YO
FOR
HEALTH

A Systematic Presentation of the Discipline of Yoga

**Institute of Naturopathy
& Yogic Sciences**

A Sterling Paperback

STERLING PAPERBACKS
An imprint of
Sterling Publishers (P) Ltd.
A-59 Okhla Industrial Area, Phase-II, New Delhi-110020.
Tel: 26387070, 26386209
Fax: 91-11-26383788 E-mail: ghai@nde.vsnl.net.in
Website: www.sterlingpublishers.com

INSTITUTE OF NATUROPATHY & YOGIC SCIENCES
Jindal Nagar, Tumkur Road, Bangalore 560073
Ph: 080-3717777 Fax: 91 3717785
E-mail: inys@satyam.net.in
www.naturecure.inys.org

Yoga for Health
© 2003, Institute of Naturopathy & Yogic Sciences
ISBN 81 207 2575 1

Published by Sterling Publishers Pvt. Ltd., New Delhi-110020.
Typeset at Vikas Compographics, New Delhi-110020.
Printed at Anandson.

Endowed with the wisdom of evenness of mind, one casts off in this life both good deeds and evil deeds; therefore, devote yourself to Yoga. Skill in action is Yoga.

Bhagavad Gita

FOREWORD

Yoga has been an integral part of our Indian culture from time immemorial. The Asanas and Kriyas, painstakingly evolved by the sages over the centuries, have been perfected to cure a wide range of diseases and also to help maintain a high standard of health. Unfortunately, many have turned a blind eye to their merits, preferring medical treatment for recovery.

Modern society the worldover, is now realising the importance of Yoga, the ancient technique of drugless therapy, after seeing the sufferings of the multitudes, due to the side effects of drugs.

The Institute of Naturopathy and Yogic Science (INYS) is endeavouring to create public awareness about this simple and natural therapy to regain and maintain physical and mental health.

Presented in this book are some important Asanas, Kriyas, Pranayama and relaxation methods and comprehensive information about their application and efficacy in treating various diseases. In order to obtain maximum benefit however, Yogic practice must be done under the guidance of a qualified and experienced teacher.

Patience and perseverance should also be exercised to achieve full benefit of Yoga. It is hoped that this book will meet the long-felt need of all those who practise Yoga and create an interest in those who have so far ignored the therapeutic values of Yoga and help them gain maximum benefit from its practice.

K R Raghunath
Chairman
INYS

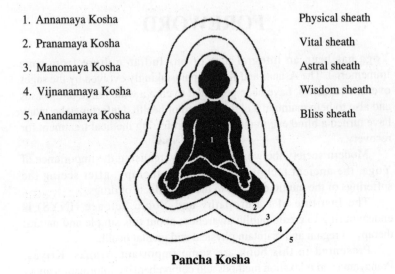

1. Annamaya Kosha	Physical sheath
2. Pranamaya Kosha	Vital sheath
3. Manomaya Kosha	Astral sheath
4. Vijnanamaya Kosha	Wisdom sheath
5. Anandamaya Kosha	Bliss sheath

Pancha Kosha

The five stages of physical existence

1. **Annamaya Kosha (Physical Sheath):** The tangible state of body. Regular yogic exercise, asanas and balanced diet can keep it healthy.

2. **Pranamaya Kosha (Vital Sheath):** The intrinsic state of body. Regular breathing exercise gives voluntary control over inhaling and exhaling which in turn keeps the 'Prana' under control.

3. **Manomaya Kosha (Astral Sheath):** The intrinsic state of body. Regular meditation, yogic sleep and prayer can pacify the mind.

4. **Vijnanamaya Kosha (Wisdom Sheath):** The intrinsic state of body. Regular self-study & enrichment of knowledge through libraries and discourses could lead towards wisdom.

5. **Anandamaya Kosha (Bliss Sheath):** The intrinsic state of body. Good deeds, self-suggested happiness and morning walk could bring us closer to this state.

PREFACE

INYS is an institution devoted to the propagation of Yoga and Naturopathy for prevention and cure of various diseases. Naturopathy and Yoga when combined, is a scientific system of medical cure, born out of observing the bio-physiological responses in human beings objectively and intimately. This system utilises and highlights nature's methods of sustenance, repair and healing with minimum interference from the outside forces. At the same time, Yoga being a complete science of life, also contributes vitality to increase the natural process in the body and in combination with Naturopathy, evolves a medical system which can give wonderful results both in case of diseases as well as, a preventive measure.

Every year thousands of patients come to INYS to learn the scientific and therapeutical aspects of Yogic Kriya, Yogasana, Pranayama, Yoga Nidra, etc., to overcome a wide-range of diseases maintain perfect health. However, it has been found that after leaving the Institute, these enthusiasts fail to practise Yoga, regularly. It must be remembered that it is by regular practice alone that full benefits of yogic science can be obtained.

The aim of writing this book is not only to remind the inmates regarding the benefits of regular Yogic practices but also to help them increase their understanding that the purpose of Yogic practices is to establish harmony between the body and mind which leads to a healthy and disease-free life.

The basic purpose of yogic management is to ensure greater efficiency in work and a better control over mind and emotions, because the various organs and systems in the body have to carry out their functions with complete coordination and harmony. If any of the organs or system fails to coordinate its functions with others, the whole system becomes imbalanced. Thus in any ailment whether physical or mental, the whole system loses coordination. Ill-health of one system creates ill-health of the other.

x

A careful study of this book and following the instructions therein will help in reaping the twin benefits of Yoga, a sound mind and a sound body. If the reader takes even one small step in achieving this significant goal, I would deem that the purpose of writing this book has been served.

Dr J J Dave
Chief Yoga Officer
INYS

CONTENTS

I

YOGA – AN INTRODUCTION

Yoga is a way to a better living. It ensures greater efficiency in work, and a better control over mind and emotions. Through Yoga one can achieve both physical and mental harmony.

It is an ancient Indian technique of integrating human personality at the physical, mental, moral and intellectual levels by means of Yogic Kriyas, Yogasanas, Pranayama, and Yoga Nidra. The aim of Yoga is to achieve a perfect balance between the individual and the cosmos. This is also a process of educating the total personality, including mental steadiness.

What is Yoga? Maharshi Patanjali defines Yoga as the control of the thought waves in the mind. Yoga is a way of life. To live a life beyond the consciousness of body, mind and intellect is its ultimate aim.

Samatvam Yoga Uchyatei, in other words, harmony or balance is Yoga.

PATHS OF YOGA

1. **Karma Yoga** – The Yoga or the act of selfless service, dedicating every work or action to God with no thought of personal reward.
2. **Bhakti Yoga** – Bhakti is undaunted love towards God, absolute surrender to the will of God. Devotion with humility, chanting, singing and repeating God's name are all important practices.
3. **Raja Yoga** – Founded by Patanjali, this is the science of physical and mental control. It is Astanga Yoga, Yoga with eight parts (limbs).
4. **Jnana Yoga** – Union with the divine through knowledge, study, thinking and meditation, using the intellect as a means to overcome bondage to the material world.

ASTANGA YOGA – The eight limbs of Yoga enumerated by Patanjali are:

1. YAMA (Social or Ethical Discipline or Restraint)

As a part of Raja Yoga, Patanjali laid emphasis on Yama, which is a symbol of social and ethical discipline, self-purification and abstinence. One of the first great commandments transcending creed, country, age and time, Yama enables one to achieve command over speech, mind, body and emotions.

(i) Ahimsa (Non-violence)

Not to kill, harm or cause any pain, either mental or physical, is the essence of Ahimsa. It is an attitude and mode of behaviour towards all living beings. The Sadhaka (the practitioner) to achieve perfection himself, keeps a watch over his mind, emotions, words and actions. A non-violent attitude is a significant aspect of a fully developed individual.

(ii) Satya (Purity of Mind)

He who speaks the truth is always courageous and not afraid of anything. Mahatma Gandhi said "Truth is God and God is Truth". Truthfulness should be practised unfolding *buddhi* (mind), perfecting it in thought, word and deed.

(iii) Asteya (Non-stealing)

Asteya means non-stealing, maintaining pure and unblemished honesty in mind and action. Stealing brings unhappiness to the person who steals. When a person practises Asteya, wealth comes to him on its own, but he may not accept it.

(iv) Brahmacharya (Celibacy)

Celibacy is a necessity for the practice of Yoga. It demands complete abstinence from sex in thought, emotion and practice. Brahmacharya is the master-key for opening the realm of health and happiness. It also consolidates vigour and strength, ensuring good health, peace and a long life.

(v) Aparigraha (Non-covetousness)

Aparigraha means non-covetousness, to keep control over one's needs. One should not desire things that are not necessary to one's life. One should cut down one's possessions and requirements to the minimum, says Patanjali. Accumulations disturbs the mind and are the root cause of all unhappiness.

2. NIYAMA (Individual Discipline)

Niyama is individual discipline, self-purification and observance of peace, both inward and outward.

(i) Sauch (Purity of Mind and Body)

Purity and cleanliness are very important for those who want to practise Yoga. Since physical purity leads to mental purity, sympathy, happiness, and good behaviour and habits are the basis for internal purification.

(ii) Tapas (Austerity)

Tapas in Sanskrit means to burn or become hot. Tapas envisages strict discipline and austerity, which helps in the purification of the mind to achieve higher levels of individual realisation. To bear pain or agony is also tapas, which purifies the sensory organs. It burns all evil and bad tendencies, controls the body and helps develop one's will power.

(iii) Santosha (Contentment)

Buddhi or intellect functions normally when the mind is peaceful. The man of santosha, satisfaction, gives up desires which brings unhappiness. Tranquillity can be achieved by practising contentment, which gives balance of mind and "Sthithapragna" qualities.

(iv) Swadhyay (Steadiness of the Self)

Regular study of religious texts in search of truth and self-realisation is Swadhyaya. Yoga Sadhaka should have both theoretical and practical knowledge of Yoga and be familiar with the literature covering its different aspects.

(v) Ishwar Pranidhan (Dedication to the Lord)

A true yogi feels that God is supreme and that he is only an instrument in His hands. Bhagavad Gita says, "whatever you do, eat, and sacrifice, whatever mortification you undergo, commit each unto Me by surrendering to me."

3. ASANA (Posture)

This brings physical as well as mental steadiness, health and vigour.

4. PRANAYAMA (Control of Breathing)

The control of the inhalation and exhalation and the retention of vital energy is called Pranayama.

5. PRATYAHARA (Control of the Mind)

Pratyahara is the control of the senses like the *shabda, sparsha, rasa, rupa* and *gandha*. This is one of the important parts of Bahiranga Yoga. This Bahiranga Yoga keeps the body strong, supple and healthy and the emotions under control. Mind is kept free from interference of senses. Pratyahara is considered to be the bridge between external and internal Yoga.

6. DHARANA (Concentration)

Complete concentration of the mind on a single point or task, for instance efforts to concentrate by remembering God or counting rosary is called Dharana.

7. DHYANA (Meditation)

Unbroken flow of thought towards God, for instance, while chanting God's name or counting rosary the string falls down, that is Dhyana.

8. SAMADHI (Superconscious State)

The state where the body and senses are at rest, as if in a sleep, but the mind and the reason alert, as if awake, is called Samadhi.

Actually Dharana, Dhyana and Samadhi are called internal (Antaranga) Yoga, as they are in close association with the mind and are ascending degree of concentration. External Yoga needs careful psycho-physical preparation of the subject.

ANTARANGA AND BAHIRANGA YOGA

Asanas improve blood circulation, digestion, excretion and respiration. Apart from that, it is one of the best forms of physical exercise, which helps in concentration and control of chitta (mind) and benefits other vital elements of the body. Since long, Pranayama is practised to control the body and the mind for achieving the pure conscious state of Yoga. By channelising the vital energy and regulating the breathing, one develops power of concentration and clarity in thinking.

In "Yoga Sutra," Patanjali broadly classified the eight limbs of Yoga as external (Bahiranga) and internal (Antaranga) Yoga. The first five of Astanga Yoga comes under Bahiranga Yoga and the last three under Antaranga Yoga.

II

PREPARATION AND PRECAUTIONS

Yoga should not be practised in a haphazard manner, without proper guidance, as it may do more harm than good. Also, not all persons should perform all the Yogic Kriyas and Asanas, hence professional expertise is necessary.

Other important requisites are the proper place, time, dress and diet, which are briefly discussed below:

1. **Place :** Select a quiet, secluded place, where fresh air is easily available like a room, verandah, terrace, garden, etc. The selected place must be free from moisture, dust, insects, bad odour and cold or hot air.

2. **Time :** Select a period of the day which suits you most. It should preferably be early hours of the morning or evening when the stomach is empty. Generally 5.00 a.m. to 8.00 a.m. is the best time for Yoga practise. The duration of practice may be fixed according to one's capacity. For instance, the duration of Pranayama may be less in the beginning but increased gradually.

3. **Dress :** Dress should be clean, light and loose-fitting to allow free movement. Light cotton garments are preferable. In cold climate a shirt or thin sweater may also be used. Remove jewellery, watch, etc., so that they do not jingle or get cut.

4. **Seat :** Since the body has to be stretched in various directions, Yogic practice must be done on a clean mat, rug, carpet or a blanket. The seat should be firm and of a good size to give comfort. Yoga must not be practised on a sofa or a soft bed.

5. **Breathing :** During Yogasana except Shitali, Shitkari and Sadanta Pranayama, inhaling and exhaling should always be through the nostrils. It should not be done through the mouth. During the

Asanas when any part of the body raises against the gravitational force, one should inhale and exhale when it comes back to the normal position. While bending forward, sideways or backwards, one should exhale. The inhaling and exhaling should be normal in the last stage of the Asana.

6. **Bath :** Bathing is not directly related to Yogasana, but a shower before, will refresh the body and mind.

7. **Food :** Yoga should be practised on an empty stomach. However, it can be practised either four hours after a heavy meal or 20 minutes after a glass of juice or a cup of skimmed milk, etc. Meals can be had half-an-hour after the practice. Avoid tea, coffee, smoking, alcohol and spices. Taking food little less than the requirements develops the elasticity in the body.

8. **Preparation of Mind :** Always begin Yoga practise with a relaxed mind. Try to keep the mind free from all disturbances and tensions. Be calm and concentrated. Observe complete silence during the practice.

9. **Illness :** Do not perform Asanas during acute illness like fever, severe asthmatic attack or extreme fatigue. Very weak patients in extreme exhaustion are warned against holding the breath (Kumbhaka) during Pranayama.

10. **In case of sinusitis, allergic cold and asthma,** soon after Jalaneti, perform Kapalbhati followed by steam inhalation.

11. **Sweating :** If there is profuse sweating during practice, do not wipe it with a towel, but rub the body with the palms, so that the temperature of the body is maintained and the process of exuding sweat continues.

12. **Sequence :** The sequence of Yogic practices, i.e. Kriyas, Asanas, Pranayama, and Yoga Nidra should be maintained.

13. **Heart Patients :** Persons suffering from heart trouble, high or low blood pressure and any serious organic disease should avoid postures which may prove dangerous. They should always be guided by doctors and Yoga experts.

14. **Professional Guidance :** Do not practise Yoga merely by studying books, seeing television or others practising it. Beginners should first take lessons from a qualified and experienced Yoga expert.

15. **Pregnancy :** Women should avoid Yogasanas, Kapalbhati, Bhastrika and Suryabhedana during menstruation. Asanas could be practised during pregnancy upto the first 80-90 days. One should not continue to do Kumbhaka and the stomach related Asanas. Pranayama could be continued throughout the pregnancy, as it helps considerably during labour. No Asana should be practised 40 to 60 days after delivery. Later, easy Asanas could be practised gradually proceeding to the usual Asanas.

16. **Diet :** Take more raw food, salad and fruits. Drink at least 8-10 glassful of water everyday. Reduce consumption of salt, sweets, spices and chillies. Avoid tea, coffee, fried food, smoking, alcohol, chewing zarda, pan masala etc.

17. **A Way of Life :** Yoga is a way of life. It must be practised regularly and conscientiously, with thorough preparation, bearing all precautions in mind for true mental and physical relaxation.

18. **O her physical exercises** like gymnastics, weightlifting, jogging, tennis, swimming, etc., should not be done immediately after Asanas and Pranayama. There should be a gap of at least 30 minutes between them.

Note

Speedy or miraculous results should not be expected immediately after starting Yoga practise. Results depend upon the individual, the nature of ailments and regularity of Yogic practice.

During the treatment period, one must be regular and try to perfect the techniques. On going home, one can perform the Yogic practices properly only after learning them correctly. Since all of them cannot be done by everybody, practice according to the prescription and requirement.

FRUITS OF YOGA

The fruits of Yoga are manifold. While it relaxes and tones up the muscles of the body, it gives total relaxation and peace to the mind.

The following are some of the major benefits derived from the practice of Yoga.

i) Vital organs get activated by systematic stimulation through various postures.

ii) It keeps the body fit and strong. It prevents diseases and prolongs life.

iii) Neuro-muscular and neuro-glandular systems get reconditioned, enabling them to withstand greater stress and strain.

iv) It increases the flexibility of the spinal cord and improves blood circulation.

v) It prevents varicose veins and piles.

vi) It tones up the abdominal organs and muscles.

vii) It reduces physical fatigue and eases menstruation.

viii) It increases secretion of gastric enzymes.

ix) It lowers triglycerides and the blood sugar level.

x) It helps in easy elimination of accumulated toxins without external aid, pressure or medication.

xi) It increases concentration by bringing better control over a wandering and wavering mind.

xii) It brings greater tranquillity to the mind and increases alertness and will power.

xiii) It helps in the cultivation of a correct mental attitude.

xiv) It gives one a feeling of health, harmony and well-being.

Regular practice of Yoga, therefore, brings about a total transformation of one's way of life. It helps in cultivating strict discipline in food habits, cleanliness, sex and character thus enabling one to become a better person.

Yoga is not only a way for upkeep of the body and mind but also a science for the health. What makes this method of treatment so powerful and effective is that it works on the principle of achieving harmony and unification in functioning the body. Realising the advantages of both, the preventive and the curative aspects of Yoga, people all over the world slowly and steadily are taking up this ancient practise. The therapeutical use of Yoga is widely known. It has become a part of our modern civilisation. The purpose of Yogic management is to establish harmony between the body and mind, which leads to a healthy and disease-free life. The Kriyas and Asanas painstakingly cultivated and developed by our sages were perfected to cure a wide range of diseases and also to maintain perfect health. Yoga is a tool to achieve a better living.

Yoga therapy comprises Yogic Kriyas, Asanas, Pranayama and Yoga Nidra or relaxation techniques etc. Let us first understand Yogic Kriyas or Shat Karma.

III

YOGIC KRIYAS – Cleansing Practices

Kriyas are a very important aspect of Hatha Yoga as they help to eliminate the accumulated toxins from the system. Neglecting those, may lead to chronic diseases. The body functions like a machine and hence has to be continuously cleaned and maintained. It is this cleansing of toxins like mucus, gas, acid, sweat, urine and stool that improves its functioning.

Kriyas help to prepare the body and condition it for the proper practice of Yogasana, Pranayama, Yoga Nidra, etc. Yogic Kriyas should always precede Asanas.

The Shat Karma – the six cleansing processes are: Neti, Dhauti, Basti, Tratak, Kapalbhati and Nauli. These Kriyas clean the eyes, respiratory system, food pipes and tone up abdominal viscera and the small intestine. They help in eliminating the toxins and morbid matter from the system. They also build up resistance to diseases, sharpen the mind and wash the colon. Apart from cleansing the system as a whole, the Kriyas also provide massaging effect on the areas applied. There are different kinds of Kriyas for cleansing the body, but the following are most important, effective and easy to practise.

1. Dhauti
2. Neti
3. Kapalbhati
4. Facial steam
5. Gargling
6. Laghu Shankh Prakshalan
7. Eye Tonic
8. Tratak

1. DHAUTI

Dhauti is a very important system of auto-cleaning. These are of many kinds but only the main types and their techniques are explained here.

a) Vastra Dhauti

Technique: This is done with a 16' long and 2" wide white muslin cloth. The cloth strip is sterilised and kept in a closed container. The sterilised strip is dipped in lukewarm water and one end is inserted deep into the mouth using the index and middle fingers. The cloth is then swallowed slowly and carefully along with the saliva. After drinking a little warm water, swallow the cloth little by little till only a small portion remains outside. Then draw out the strip slowly with both the hands. The whole process should not exceed 20 minutes.

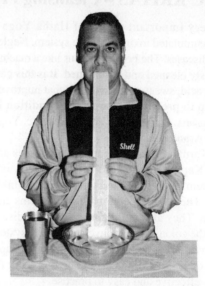

Vastra Dhauti

Important Points

1. Practice this Kriya on an empty stomach only.
2. Remove the strip within 20 minutes of insertion.
3. Do not speak during the practice.
4. If the practitioner experiences difficulty, lukewarm water may be given to drink.

5. If there is a tendency to itch, stop for a while and continue insertion after itching stops.

6. Do not perform this Kriya without expert guidance.

Limitations: Persons suffering from gastric and duodenal ulcers, hypertension, heart problems and hernia should not practise this Kriya.

Frequency: Normally once in a week, but can be done more depending on circumstances.

Benefits: Help in the treatment of asthma, bronchitis, chronic cough and other respiratory disorders. Removes the excessive bile and phlegm from stomach. It is a good remedy for indigestion and dyspeptic conditions.

b) Vamana Dhauti or Kunjal

Technique: Take lukewarm water (44°C) flavoured with aniseed and cardamom. While sitting in Kagasana (as shown in the picture) drink four to six glasses of water or as much as possible in quick succession till vomiting sensation is felt. Stand up immediately, bend forward and insert the first three fingers of the right hand into far back of the mouth and tickle till vomiting takes place. The water will gush out of the mouth. Continue the process till all the water comes out and the stomach becomes empty.

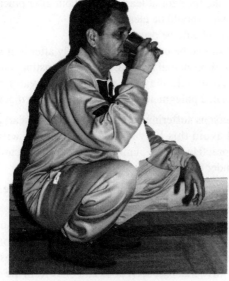

Vamana Dhauti (a)

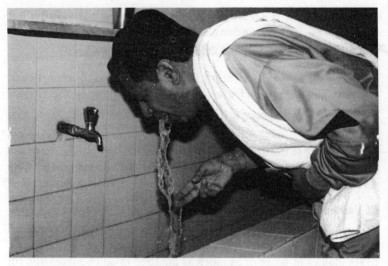

Vamana Dhauti (b)

Important Points

1. Practise Vamana Dhauti in the early morning on an empty stomach.
2. Do not take food for at least half-an-hour after practice.
3. Finger nails should be clean and cut.
4. The water should be drunk quickly.
5. Jalaneti should be practised immediately after it, if necessary.
6. In cases of bronchial asthma, diabetes, constipation, arthritis and gas, a little salt may be added to the water to expel the accumulated phlegm and other toxins from the digestive system.

Limitations: Persons suffering from stom, ii ulcers, heart problems and hernia should avoid this Kriya. However, patients with high blood pressure may practise it with plain ater, or aniseed, cardamom water without salt, under expert gu. iance.

Fr   ncy: Norr al'y once a week, but more often in special cir.   :es.

?e η   : Highly recommended for patients suffering from indigestion, astaina, diabete., constipation, chronic cold and nervous weakness. Va. ina ' ya cleanses the upper portion of gastro-intestinal tract by remov excessive mucosal secretions and biles from the system.

2. NETI

Neti means cleansing of nostrils. This is of two kinds.
- a) Sutraneti / Rubberneti
- b) Jalaneti

Ghee Drops

Before doing Sutraneti and Jalaneti put a few drops of warm ghee (50 to 54°C) into each nostril while in the supine position. This lubricates and eases elimination of mucous through the nostril. After putting ghee, cover the face with a folded towel and press the area around the nose.

a) Sutraneti / Rubberneti

Technique: Traditionally, a cotton string stiffened with wax was used for this purpose. But now-a-days, a thin rubber catheter of 3, 4 or 5 numbers is generally used. The rounded portion of the string or tube is inserted through one nostril down the throat and pulled out through the mouth with the help of the first and middle fingers of the left hand. Then both the ends are pulled to and fro so that it moves backward and forward in the nostril. Do this 15 to 20 times. Remove the string through the mouth and repeat the same procedure for the other nostril.

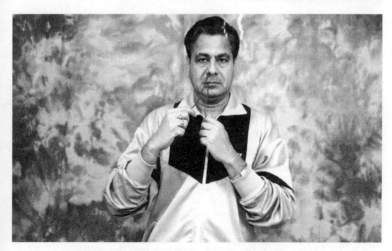

Sutraneti

Important Points

1. The Sutraneti or the rubber catheter should be pushed through the nostrils gently and slowly.

2. Finger nails should be cut properly before doing this Kriya.

3. Spectacles (if any) should be removed before practising.

4. In the first few practices, when the thread or catheter is introduced into the nose, there might be an itching or irritating sensation in the nostrils which may cause sneezing. The eyes may also water, but these symptoms will subside with regular practice.

Frequency: Once in the morning, daily, to be followed by Jalaneti. This should be practised twice a week after 3 to 4 months.

Limitations: Persons suffering from haemorrhage in the nose and acute cold should not practise this without guidance.

Benefits: It opens up blocked nasal passages and gives relief during throat ailment. It toughens the nasal mucus and renders them less sensitive to irritation of dust particles. It is also very useful in cases of migraine, sinusitis and asthma. It increases the oxygen intake into the lungs and improves the working efficiency of respiratory system.

b) Jalaneti (Nasal Douche)

Jalaneti is another technique of nasal cleansing. Here the cleansing is done by salt water.

Technique: This requires a special type of vessel (Neti Lota) which has a spout. Boil a pot of water and allow it to cool till it becomes lukewarm (upto 42°C). Add a teaspoonful of salt and stir well. Stand erect, stoop forward and insert the spout gently into one of the nostrils. Slowly tilt the head to the other side so that the water runs into one nostril and comes out through the other. Keep the mouth open and breathe normally through the mouth. Allow the water to flow freely through the other nostril continuously like a stream. Repeat the process with the other nostril.

Important Points

1. The concentration of salt and the temperature of the water should be maintained throughout the practice.

2. Do not insert the nozzle too much into the nostril.

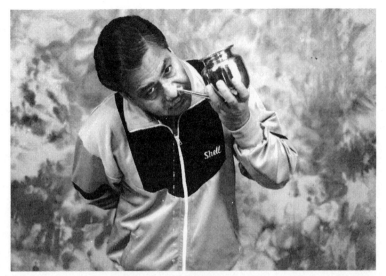

Jalaneti

3. During the practice do not inhale through the nose or else the salt water will go inside the mouth.

4. Initially, when water enters the nose, there could be an itching or irritating sensation causing sneezing. But with repeated practice these symptoms will cease.

5. The nose should be dried properly after Jalaneti. Any water left may cause cold and sinusitis. Drying of nose can be done by bending in all directions and exhaling forcefully.

Frequency: Must be practised in the morning, daily, if one is suffering from cold and stuffy nose for 3 to 4 months, thereafter twice a week.

Benefits

1. Cleans the upper respiratory tract by removing mucosal secretions, making respiration smooth and easy. Also improves the functional efficiency of the mucous membrane and olfactory nerves.

2. Gives relief from sore throat, nasal catarrh, cold, cough, sinusitis, migraine, headache and inflammation of the nasal membranes.

3. Gives a cooling and soothing effect to the brain and is helpful in depression.

4. Helps in doing Pranayama easily as the nasal passage becomes clear and respiration easy and smooth after Jalaneti.

3. KAPALBHATI

After completing Jalaneti, exhalation to dry the nose should be done. Ensure that Kapalbhati is done in a standing position, keeping the legs apart and both the hands at the back. Bend forward and quickly exhale water through the nostrils. Move the neck forward, backward and to the left and right. Exhalation should be forceful and vigorous and should be accompanied by a hissing sound. It also can be performed in a sitting position.

4. FACIAL STEAM

Exhalation is essential if some water remains inside the nasal cavity, specially for people suffering from sinusitis, cold, cough, bronchitis, allergic rhinitis and asthma. Steam inhalation with a few leaves or few drops of eucalyptus oil for a few minutes will be very helpful. This should be followed by Kapalbhati and ghee drops. The nose should be properly dried (by pinching the nasal passage if necessary) to make respiration easy and smooth.

5. GARGLING

Gargle with warm water (52°C approx.) to which 2 to 3 per cent salt has been added. This will help in cleansing the throat, removing excessive mucus and irritation. Doing so regularly also improves one's voice. In case of burning sensation or pain in the throat, add a spoonful of honey to warm water and gargle with it. Gargling also activates thyroid gland.

6. LAGHU SHANKHA PRAKSHALANA (LSP)

This is irrigation of the entire alimentary tract with water. The alimentary passages are very tortuous and the exit is very narrow like a conch (shankh). Since this is washed in this Kriya, the ancients gave this process an appropriate name – Shankha Prakshalana.

Here Laghu Shankha Prakshlana is explained which is easier, comfortable and eliminates the toxins from the system. While sitting in Kagasana drink two glasses of lukewarm water (44° to 45°C) with rock salt (in 6 glasses of water add 2 tsp. rock salt or seadha rapzak) in three phases. After every two glasses of water, perform the Asanas mentioned below in the given sequence, five times on each side. This helps ease the passage of water and flush the intestines more briskly. Within 15 to 30 minutes one gets an urge to evacuate the bowels. Try to do so without strain for a minute. After this, the patient usually will have clear bowel movement and discharge large quantity of urine.

After Laghu Shankha Prakshalana, there is restriction on diet, treatment, Yogasana etc. One should take proper meals after 4 hours and it should be simple without salt and masalas. Eat simply cooked *khichari* (dish made of rice and pulses) with clarified butter.

It is dangerous to do this Kriya frequently. This may be practised once a month. It is advisable to avoid other Kriyas after this. Just lie down in Shavasana for 5 to 10 minutes and relax yourself.

Sequence of the Asanas

A. Tadasana
B. Triyaka Tadasana
C. Kati Chakrasana
D. Triyaka Bhujangasana
E. Udarakarshasana

A. Tadasana (Up-stretched Pose)

Stand erect with both the hands close to the body. Inhale, rise on the toes and lift the arms above the head by intertwining the fingers. Exhale, lower the arms and stand flat on the feet. Do this 10 times.

B. Triyaka Tadasana (Side-stretched Pose)

Stand erect, keep the legs apart, raise the hands up, parallel to the ears. Intertwine the fingers with palms facing upwards. While exhaling, bend laterally. Return to the normal position. Inhale without bending the knees and the arms. Repeat it on the opposite side. Do this five times on each side.

C. Kati Chakrasana (Spinal Twist)

Stand erect, keep the legs apart. Stretch the arms at shoulder level. Twist the upper part of the body towards the right shoulder keeping left palm over right shoulder and wrap the right arm around the trunk in a smooth motion. Repeat this on the opposite side by changing the position of hands. Do this exercise five times on each side, breathing should be normal.

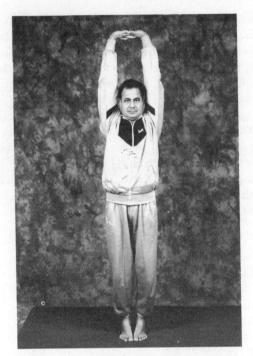

Tadasana

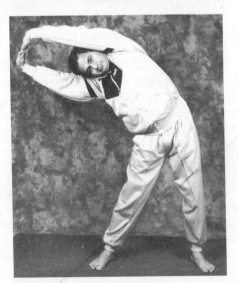

Triyaka Tadasana

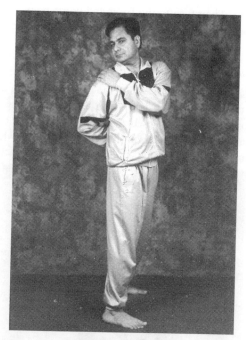

Kati Chakrasana

D. Triyaka Bhujangasana (Twisted Cobra Pose)

Lie down in prone position. Place hands on the side of the chest and legs apart. While inhaling raise the head, chest and abdomen. Rest on the palms, then twist to right side from the waist upwards, looking to left heel

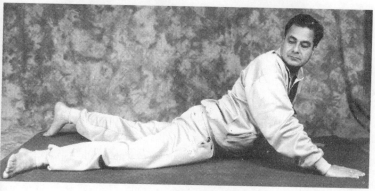

Triyaka Bhujangasana

while exhaling. Then turn to the front and come back to the original position. Repeat the process on the left side. Do this five times on each side.

E. Udarakarshasana (Belly Section Pose)

Sit in Utkatasana posture (as shown in the picture) keeping the palms on the knees on the respective sides. While exhaling, lower one of the knees to touch the opposite toe and slowly turn your whole upper body towards the side of that toe. Then come back slowly to Utkatasana while inhaling. Repeat the same on the other side. Do this five times on each side.

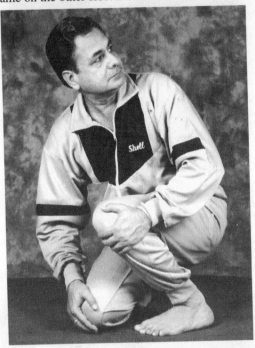

Udarakarshasana

Important Points of Laghu Shankha Prakshalana

1. This Kriya should be done in the morning on an empty stomach.

2. Take only rock salt (in 6 glasses of water add 2 tsp. rock salt or sendha namak).

3. Wear light and comfortable clothes.

4. This should be practised in a relaxed mood and without tension or trepidation.

5. Evacuate the bowels without strain.

6. Do not worry if a longer time is taken to evacuate or if you have to drink more water than the others.

7. This Kriya should be performed under expert guidance only. It should not be practised repeatedly.

8. It should not be done during fasting, sickness and menstruation period.

Limitations: Persons suffering from high blood pressure, gastric or duodenal ulcers, piles and ulcerative colitis should avoid this Kriya.

Benefits: Laghu Shankha Prakashalana cleanses the whole alimentary passages and is highly recommended for persons suffering from chronic constipation, gas, acidity, indigestion, diabetes, asthma and other digestive and respiratory disorders. It is also good for the kidney and urinary systems as it helps prevent urinary infection.

7. NATURAL EYE TONIC (for external use only)

Composition

Amla	40%
Harade	25%
Baheda	20%
Chandan Powder	11%
Parch Karpoor	4%
(Edible Camphor)	

Procedure for Use

Soak half a teaspoonful of natural eye tonic powder overnight in 200 ml of water in a glass or an earthern pot. Next morning filter it and this is ready for use.

First, wash the eye-cups and fill it with the prepared eye tonic. Holding the eye-cups in the hand, bend the head so that the eyeball touches the tonic. Blink 30 to 40 times slowly. Wash the eye-cup (to avoid infection).

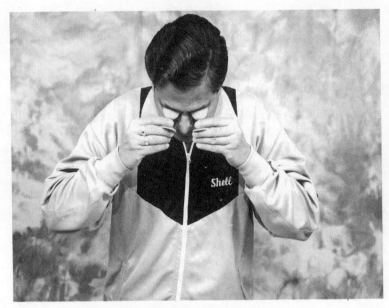

Cleansing the Eye with Eye Tonic

Benefits: Cleanses the eye thoroughly, relieves tension in the eyeballs and soothes watery and sore eyes. Useful in treating myopia, hypermetropia, presbyopia and headache. Improves eyesight, increases blood supply to the eyes and the optic nerves.

8. TRATAKA AND PALMING

Trataka

Trataka is an eye exercise which is done by focusing the eye on a selected object.

Technique : Sit in a comfortable meditative posture with head, neck, and back erect and the body relaxed. Place an object (a burning candle or a small lamp) at eye level, at a distance of around one meter from the face. Close the eyes. Be aware of the physical body and be still like a statue. Then open the eyes and gaze intently at the spot or the brightest spot of the flame just above the wick.

Continue gazing at the spot of the flame with total concentration without moving the eyeball, or blinking. Forget the body and centre the whole concentration on the eyes. When the eyes get tired or tears come out, close the eyes and relax. Be aware of the after image of the flame in front of the closed eyes. As it fades, open the eyes and again concentrate on the flame. Repeat this 3 to 5 times, then close the eyes and then relax completely.

Important Points

1. This Kriya should be practised under guidance only.
2. The body should not be moved throughout the practice.
3. The eyes should not be blinked nor the eyeballs moved during the practice.
4. If a lighted lamp or candle is used, then practise in a closed room where the flame will be steady and is not affected by a drought of air.

Limitations: Persons having glucoma or chronic eye disorders should seek medical advice before practising it.

Frequency: It can be done at any time, but preferabl y during early morning and late night, daily for 15 to 20 minutes.

Palming

Sit comfortably, close the eyes, gently rub your palms and cover them with the palms in such a way as to avoid any pressure on the eyeballs and without allowing light to pass through. If it is not completely dark before the eyes during palming, and some other colour appears, it indicates that the eyes and mind are under strain. This may be practised for minimum 2 to 3 minutes.

Note: Also do Trataka and take Facial Steam (Vapour) followed by Shavasana.

Benefits: This is one of the best exercises for removing tension, fatigue and myopia. Regular practice improves eyesight. It is a very good exercise for the eye muscles and the optic nerves.

SEQUENCE OF KRIYAS

1. Vastra Dhauti
2. Vamana Dhauti

3. Ghee drops in the nostrils
4. Rubber / Sutraneti
5. Jalaneti
6. Kapalbhati / Exhalation exercises and facial steam
7. Gargling
8. Laghu Shaukha Prakashalana
9. Eye tonic

(Above- mentioned Kriyas should be practised after consulting a doctor or a Yoga expert.)

IV

SURYANAMASKAR

Suryanamaskar is the ancient ritual of saluting the sun. It also limbers up the body.

Suryanamaskar has an important place in Yogasana and it offers innumerable benefits as it is Asana, Pranayama and Bandha, all combined.

There are many types of Suryanamaskars. Of all these, the simplest one is described below. Twelve poses constitute one Suryanamaskar. One must move from one pose to the other in a continuous motion.

Technique

Pose 1: Stand erect, keeping legs together and knees straight (back of the head should be in line with the rest of the body). In Namaskar Mudra, fold

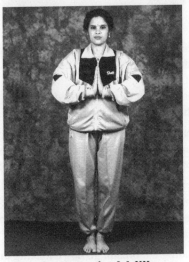

Suryanamaskar I & XII

the arms and bring the hands in front of the chest. Thumbs must touch the middle of the chest and forearms be kept outward and stiff and the eyes closed. Breathing should be normal.

Pose 2: Open the eyes and while inhaling, raise the arms. Bend backwards from the waist without bending the knees.

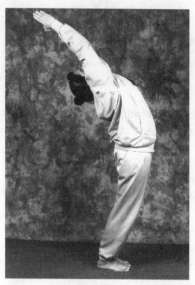

II & XI

Pose 3: While exhaling, slowly bend forward and try to touch the ground without bending the knees. If possible, keep the palms by the side of the feet on the ground.

In the beginning it may be difficult to do so, but by practice one can achieve this. Further, try to touch the forehead to the knees.

Pose 4: While inhaling, move the right leg back, as far as possible. Then keeping the toes and knee of the right leg on the ground, raise the head, bend your spine backward and look upward. The left leg should remain flexed at the knee, the palms flat on the ground in line with the left foot.

Pose 5: While exhaling, move the left leg back like the right leg, toes and knee touching the ground. Now raise the complete body, like a sloping plank with palms and toes touching the ground.

Pose 6: While holding the breath, go down making the forehead, chest, palms, knees and toes touch the ground, but not the abdomen. This is

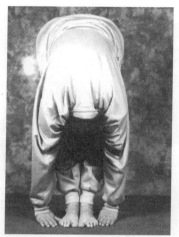

III & X

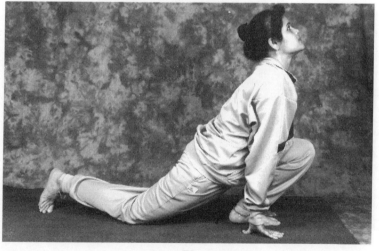

IV

called Sastang Namaskar. In the initial stages, there may be some difficulty, but gradually one can learn the pose.

Pose 7: While inhaling, raise the front part of the body supported by the palms and bend backwards to the maximum with eyes looking towards the sky. In this pose, the knees must touch the ground.

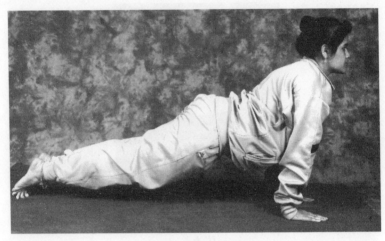

V

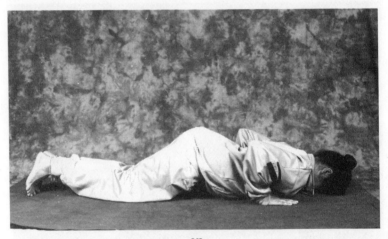

VI

Pose 8: While exhaling, raise the complete body backward and upward like a pyramid, keeping the feet fully on the ground. The head must be in between the shoulders, chin touching the jugular notch in such a way that the navel is in view.

Pose 9: While inhaling bring right leg forward and between the hands. This position resembles the fourth pose.

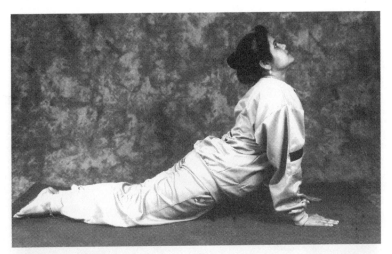

VII

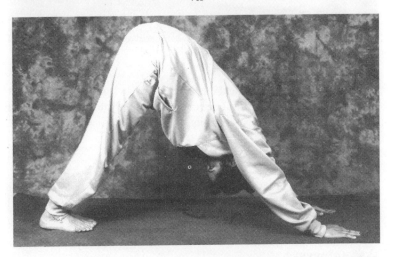

VIII

Pose 10: Bring the left leg forward upto the right foot. While exhaling, bend forward and try to touch the ground without bending at the knees. This position is Padahastasana as in third pose.

Pose 11: Raise both the arms straight up while inhaling and bend backward without bending at the knees, as in pose no. 2.

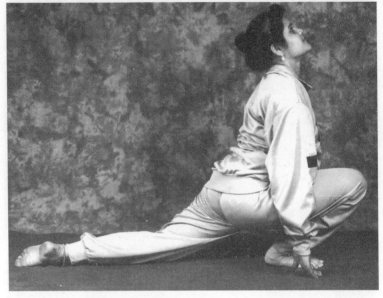

IX

Pose 12: While exhaling, stand erect with palms in front of the chest, just as in the first pose. This constitutes one round of Suryanamaskar. One can do as many as ones capacity permits.

Warning

It should not be practised by patients suffering from severe lumbar spondylosis, inflamed joints, hypertension, cardiac disorders, ulcer and vertigo. Also avoid in case of hernia and renal disorder.

Advantages

It gives combined benefits of Asanas, Pranayama and exercise. Pose no. 4 and 9 give good exercise to the spleen and liver. The other poses exercise lungs, intestines and kidneys. By regular practice of Suryanamaskar, the body will always be active and functions of the organs will improve. It is beneficial in cases of bronchial asthma, diabetes mellitus, initial stage of arthritis, irregular menstruation and constipation. It also improves vitality.

V

YOGASANAS

Yoga is a way to better living. It ensures greater efficiency in work, better control over mind and emotions. Through Yoga, one can achieve both physical fitness and mental harmony.

Asanas, an intrinsic part of Yoga, are body postures designed to harmoniously blend mind and body to achieve complete physical and mental relaxation. Regular practice of Yogasana rejuvenates the entire physiological system. Yogasana postures, in fact, help the body in maintaining good health by improving its ability to resist diseases.

Asanas work mainly on the endocrine and nervous systems. Since both these systems are inter-related, the effects produced on these two reflect on the other systems as well.

HOW ASANAS ARE DIFFERENT FROM BODY EXERCISE

Asanas and exercise should not be done together because they are not complimentary to each other. Energy is restored after practising Asanas while energy is exhausted by doing the exercise. Hence one feels fresh and energetic after doing the Asanas but feels tired after the exercise. Internal organs get the benefit of massage while practising Asanas, while muscles become strong by doing the exercise. The elasticity of the body is increased with the Asanas whereas exercise makes body hard. The person practising the Asanas always looks stable, strong and young. It effects not only the body but also the *mana* (the inner self) and one experiences the peace and stability. Exercise only affects the body.

TIPS FOR PERFORMING ASANAS CORRECTLY

1. One can drink water or fruit juice half an hour before and after practising Yoga.

2. Asanas should always be performed with concentration and at ease, slowly and gradually taking care of the proper breathing.

3. In breathing one must remember that inhale while your hand or feet goes against the gravitational force (above the ground) and exhale, when you come back to the normal position. In between, breathing should be normal. When you turn your body or bend (forward, or to the back), exhale. Inhale when you come back to the normal position. In between breathing should be normal.

4. While practising the Asanas always give importance to exhale as much as you can. This will give more benefit.

5. Always practice Asanas twice (doing left and right both sides means once).

6. Maintain the Asana posture as long as possible and gradually increase the time.

7. Avoid jerky movements while assuming or releasing the Asanas.

8. Ensure that the correct posture is assumed and retained for a correct period.

9. Study the accompanying photographs thoroughly to get the correct posture.

10. Understand the purpose of each Asana so that while retaining it, concentration can be bestowed on the particular organ to be exercised.

11. Starting from the easy postures go to the more difficult ones. Number of Asanas can be reduced or increased for the patients depending on the diagnose, age, vitality and ability of the patients.

YOGASANAS FOR HEALTHY LIVING

Asana I	Asana II	Asana III	Asana IV
	Ardha Halasana		
Ardha Halasana	Uttan Padasana	Suryanamaskar	Suryanamaskar
Ardha Pavan M.	Pagachalana		Vipareet Karni
Uttan Tadasana	Pavan Muktasana	Halasana	Suptavajrasana

Katichalana	Sethubandhasana	Matsyasana	Bhujangasana
	Bhujangasana	Utthit Padasana	Shalabhasana
Parvatasana	Ardha Shalabhasana	Triyak Bhujangasana	Dhanurasana
		Shalabhasana	
Vakrasana	Hastha Parshwasana	Janusirasana	Paschimottanasana
Gomukhasana	Vakrasana	Ardha Matsyendrasana	Ustrasana
Shavasana	Shavasana	Mandukasana	Shashankasana
		Shirshasana	Shirshasana
		Shavasana	Shavasana

SUKSHMA VYAYAMA

Tadasana, Chakrasana, Kati Chakrasana and neck, shoulder, ankle, eye, and abdominal exercise.

Additional Asanas

(i) Skandha Katiasana, Kati Shakti, Merudanda Shithilikarna, Cross Katichalan, Ardha Dhanurasana, Sarpasana, Naukasana.

(ii) Pranayama: Suryabhedana, Chandrabhedan, Sadanta, Shitali, Shitakari, Ujjayi.

Infact regular practice of Yogasana goes a long way in controlling various diseases and improving physical fitness, flexibility of various joints by removing stiffness, increasing immunity and toning up the functioning abilities of organs like kidney, lung, intestine, liver and skin. Asanas also help in breaking down of excess fat, and increases blood circulation. It increases the coronary blood flow, oxygen assimilation and eases the flow of pranic energy to the whole body. Asanas could be practised by individuals depending on the age, capacity and the disease to be treated. They should be performed on an empty stomach. Final position should be maintained with deep and slow breathing. The time limit of retaining final posture depends on one's capacity, which will be increased gradually. Start with a simple posture and then take up more difficult ones.

Warning: Practising Yoga in a wrong manner or method will not bestow any benefit, but may prove harmful. Therefore, guidance of an expert and an experienced teacher is a must.

SUPINE POSES

SHAVASANA (Corpse or Relaxation Pose)

Lie flat on the back, feet comfortably apart, arms and hands extended about 6" away from the body, palms facing upwards with half-folded fingers. Close the eyes. Now gently relax the feet, keeping them completely still. Then relax the knees, then the chest and the arms. Keep both the hands still to achieve a relaxed position. Concentrate next on the head. Move it gently to the side, let it rest and keep it free from all thoughts. Then concentrate the mind on rhythmic breathing. The abdomen should come out while inhaling and go inside while exhaling. Breathing should be as slow and effortless as possible. Thus all the parts of the body are loosened to create a state of complete relaxation. This relaxed position should be maintained for 10 to 15 minutes.

Benefits: It helps to bring down high blood pressure (arterial hypertension) and gives immense relief to the mind, particularly for those engaged in mental activity like reading and writing. This Asana could be

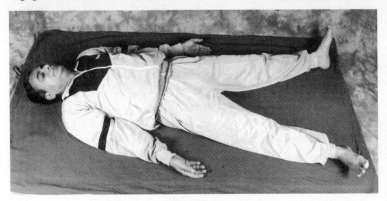

Shavasana

performed even by those who are advised against doing other Asanas due to high blood pressure. It helps ease tension and stress for those involved in physical activities. This Asana should be performed after completing the daily round of Yogic Asanas. Shavasana done during fasting soothes the nervous system.

ARDHA HALASANA

Lie on the back with feet together. Keep your palms beside the thighs, facing the ground. Now inhale and raise the right leg, as much as possible, without bending the knee. Be in the posture for sometime, breathe normally and while exhaling bring the leg down slowly. Then repeat the Asana with the left leg.

Benefits: This Asana gives an excellent exercise to the pelvic region. Any pain in the lumbar region due to wrong posture or pressure could be rectified to a great extent by its regular practice. It also burns the excess fat in the thighs, hips and abdomen.

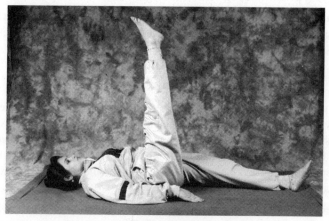

Ardha Halasana

UTTAN PADASANA (Leg Raising)

Lie on the back with legs and arms straight, feet together, palms facing ground and touching the sides of the body. While inhaling gradually raise the legs to 30°, 60° and then to 90°, pausing slightly at each angle without

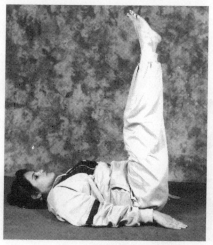

Uttan Padasana

bending the knees. At the 90° position, raise the toes upwards while body lies on the ground from the head to coccyx. Maintain this posture for sometime and breathe normally. Then, while exhaling, slowly go back to the lying position through the same stages without bending the knees.

Benefits: Helpful in curing nervous weakness and constipation. Strengthens abdominal muscles and intestinal organs. Avoid in severe back and knee pain.

UTTHIT PADASANA (Balancing Pose)

Lie on the back with legs outstretched. The hands should be beside the hips. Now, while inhaling, raise the body above the hips and below the waist, as far as possible from the ground. Raise the hands from the ground and bring them to the side of the thighs. Hold this posture for a while, breathe normally and then return back slowly to the lying position while exhaling.

Benefits: Utthit Padasana is essential for maintaining the navel in its normal position. Any displacement of the navel results in a variety of abdominal disorders such as pain, flatulence, indigestion, diabetes, etc. For restoring a displaced navel to its original position and to prevent it from further displacement, Utthit Padasana is extremely useful.

Warning: Persons suffering from ulcers and lumbar spondylosis should not perform this Asana.

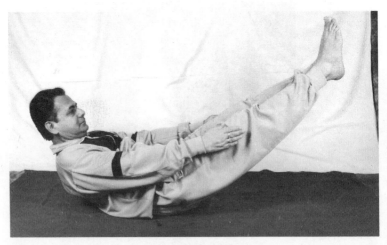

Utthit Padasana

SARVANGASANA (Shoulder Stand)

This Asana is very good for the thyroid gland. Lie on the back with legs and arms straight, feet together and palms on the floor beside the body. While inhaling, raise the legs slowly upto 90° and then the whole body, and rest the weight on the arms so that the chin touches the jugular notch. Bring the arms and hands to support the body at the hip region (fingers at the back and thumb in front of the body). The entire weight of the body rests on the head, neck and shoulders while the arms are used for balancing. Keep the trunk, legs and hips in a straight line and as vertical as possible. Focus the eyes on the big toes, with the chin pressed against the chest. Retain the posture for one to three minutes and breathe normally. While exhaling, return to lying position by bringing the leg backward and releasing the hands and the palms.

Benefits: Improves the activities of reproductive organs in both men and women. Helps in relieving bronchitis, dyspepsia, varicose veins and

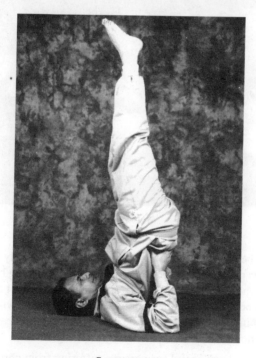

Sarvangasana

increases digestive capacity. It stimulates the thyroid and para-thyroid glands and influences the brain, heart and lungs. Improves blood circulation and quietens the mind.

Warning: This posture should not be practised by those suffering from high blood pressure.

MATSYASANA (Fish Pose)

This Asana is called Matsyasana because a person can float on water like a fish for sometime if he lies in this posture while swimming. Sit with legs fully stretched out. Bend one after another legs at the knees and place the feet on the other hip joint. Adjust both the heels are in such a way that each presses the adjacent portion of the abdomen. This forms the foot-lock in a sitting position. Bend backwards while exhaling and rest your

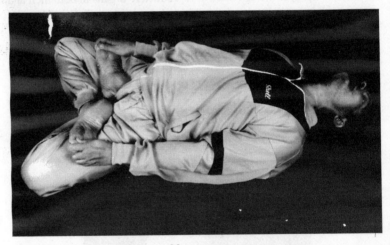

Matsyasana

weight on the elbows. Push the neck backward and slightly rise the hip upward thus making an arch of the spine. Then, by making hooks of the forefingers, hold the toes on the corresponding side without crossing the arms. This posture should be maintained for some time with slow and deep breathing. For reverting to the original position, release the foot-lock and return to the supine position by lowering the arch.

Benefits: It is very useful for persons suffering from chronic cough, bronchial asthma, congestion, infected tonsils and other respiratory disorders. Problems relating to thyroid and para-thyroid glands could also be overcome by performing this Asana.

Matsyasana should be done to derive full benefits of Sarvangasana.

SUPTAVAJRASANA (Supine Thunderbolt Pose)

Sit with both legs folded and placed under the hips. Let the heels touch the hips with toes touching each other. Slowly part the legs in such a way that hips rest between the feet. Then tilt backwards resting the elbows one by one behind. Gradually rest the shoulders and the head flat on the ground. Then stretch your hands upwards and make a cushion under the head.

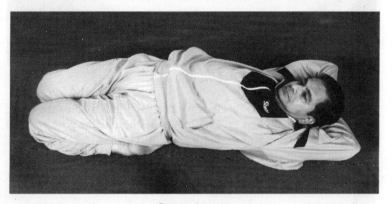

Suptavajrasana

Breathing should be normal. Retain the posture for some time and then return to the normal sitting position in a reverse order.

Benefits: This is one of the useful variations of Matsyasana. It is helpful in treating ailments of the neck, back and waist. It makes the spine resilient and streamlines the abdomen.

Warnings: Persons suffering from severe pain in knee joints or with slipped disc and lumbago should avoid Suptavajrasana.

HALASANA (Plough Pose)

Lie flat on the back with legs and feet together, arms at the sides and placed beside the thighs. Keeping the legs straight, while inhaling slowly, raise them to 30°, 60° and then to 90° slightly pausing at each stage. While exhaling push the legs further over and above the head and then beyond, so that the toes touch the floor (without bending the knees). Stretch the

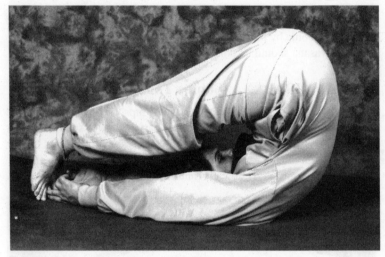

Halasana

legs as far as possible so that the chin presses tightly against the chest. Then raise the hands and try to hold the toes. Retain the pose from 10 seconds to 3 minutes. Breathe normally while inhaling.

Straighten the legs while exhaling, return to the starting position.

Precaution: Hernia, high blood pressure, ulcer and cervical spondylosis patients should avoid this Asana.

Benefits: Improves digestion and strengthens the spine. Helps in asthma, diabetes, menstrual disorder and constipation.

ARDHA PAVAN MUKTASANA (Simple)

Lie down on the back with the feet close together. Place the palms beside the body. Inhale, raise the right leg and bend it at the knee. Bring the thigh near the abdomen, interlock the fingers, while exhaling press the thigh against the abdomen and hold the posture for few seconds. Breathe normally. While inhaling, stretch the leg up and while exhaling, bring the leg back on the floor. Repeat the same with the left leg. Except high blood pressure, heart-related problems and cervical spondylosis, one can raise the head and touch the chin to the knees.

Benefits: This Asana is very helpful in removing the gases accumulated in the digestive tract. It is good for pains of back, abdomen and buttocks. It smoothens the functions of liver, spleen, stomach, kidney and pancreas.

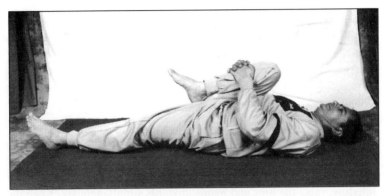

Ardha Pavan Muktasana

PAVAN MUKTASANA (Gas Releasing Pose) (Simple)

Keep the hands by the side of the body in the supine position. While inhaling, raise both the legs upto 90° and bend them at the knees. Make a finger lock with both the hands around them, a little below the knees. While exhaling, bring the thighs close to the chest by contracting the abdominal muscles. Maintain this posture for a few seconds, breathe normally. Then return to the original posture in the reverse order as Ardha Pavan Muktasana. Repeat the Asana twice. Except high blood pressure, heart-related problems and cervical spondylosis, one can raise the head and touch the chin to the knees.

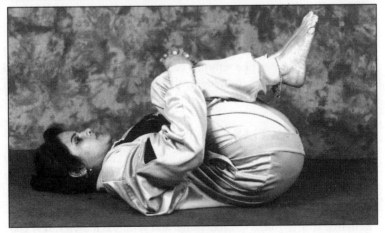

Pavan Muktasana

Benefits: Pavan Muktasana strengthens the abdominal muscles and organs like the liver, spleen, pancreas and stomach. It releases excess gas from the abdomen. Persons suffering from constipation must do this after drinking lukewarm water for proper evacuation of bowels in the morning. Pavan Muktasana is the best Asana to expel gas by compression of the abdomen.

SETUBANDHASANA (Bridge Pose)

Lie down in Shavasana posture. Raise the knees and bring the feet nearer to the hips, keeping them apart. Keep the hands near the thighs. While inhaling, raise the hips and hands upwards simultaneously. Keep the hands over the head on the floor, breathe normally. Bring back the hands and hips to the original position while exhaling. Repeat twice and relax.

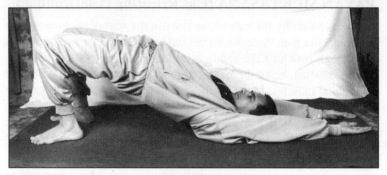

Setubandhasana

Benefits: Regular practice of this Asana is helpful in mitigating painful conditions in diseases like arthritis, cervical or lumbar spondylosis and sciatica. This also helps in strengthening the muscles of the chest, hips, shoulders and hands.

SKANDHA KATIASANA

Lie on your back gently, bend both the legs at the knees and bring the feet near the hips. While inhaling, slowly raise hands and shoulders and try to touch the knees. Retain the posture for few seconds. Breathe normally. While exhaling return to the starting position.

Benefits: It strengthens the abdominal and vertebral muscles. It is good for arthritis, stiff back, respiratory disorder, diabetes and constipation.

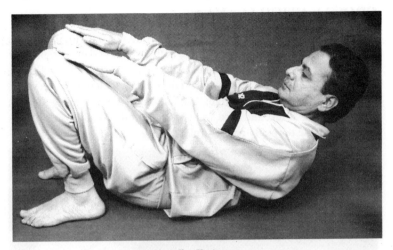

Skandha Katiasana

KATICHALANA (Spine Twisting Pose)

Lie flat on the back, bend both the legs at the knees and bring the feet near the hips. Interlock the fingers of both the hands and keep them under the head.

Now exhale and give a little pressure on the waist. Twist your knees to the right, simultaneously turning head and neck to the left. Maintain normal breathing. Again, while exhaling, twist the knees to the left, turning the head and neck to the right, breathe normally. Repeat this twice on each side. Come back to the normal position and then relax.

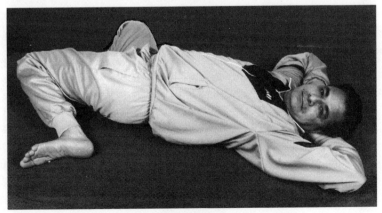

Katichalana

CROSS KATICHALANA

Similar to Katichalana – Cross leg twisting pose, lie in Shavasana, bring the legs and hands together. Fold both the legs and cross right over the left. Interlock fingers of both the hands and keep under the head. Now, while exhaling, twist the leg towards right and look at left and vice versa. Change the leg, left over the right. While exhaling, twist the leg towards right and look at left and vice versa. Maintain the final position for a minute, breathe normally and return in reverse order.

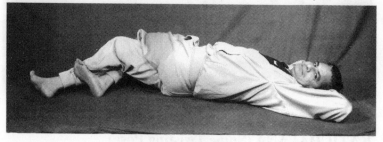

Cross Katichalana

Benefits: Very good in relieving back pain and also helps in digestion and joint pains.

It maintains the flexibility of spine and also gives good exercise to the abdomen, hips, chest, knees, shoulder and spine. It also relieves joint pains and helps in curing diabetes and constipation.

PAGACHALANA (Leg Twisting Pose)

Lie down flat on your back and stretch your hands sideways to your shoulder with palms on the floor. Now keep the heel of the right leg between the big and small toe of the left foot. Keep both the feet erect, one upon the other in this position. Now, without changing the position of your feet, while exhaling try to touch the right foot to the ground on the left side. While turning your head to the right and vice versa, stay in the position for some time. The same should be repeated, by keeping the left foot over the right. Breathing should be normal. Do this exercise twice with each leg and then rest in Shavasana for a while.

Benefits: This exercise is a variation of Katichalana and is very useful in relieving pain in the back, legs and shoulders. Pancreas and liver become strong. It also renders the body supple and agile.

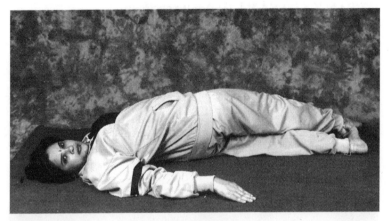

Pagachalana

KATISHAKTIASANA

Lie on your back gently. Keep your legs slightly apart. Clasp hands over your chest. While inhaling, try to touch both the toes by tilting the pelvis. Retain in final pose. Exhale and come back to the starting position. Breathe normally.

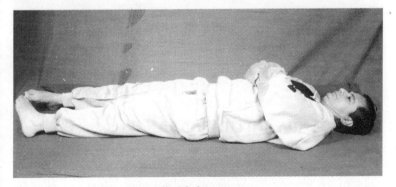

Katishaktiasana

Benefits: It is a good exercise for sciatica pain, hip joints pain, lumbar spondylosis and also relieves stiffness of lower back, thighs, calves and feet.

UTTAN TADASANA (Palm Tree Pose)

Lie on the back and join the feet such that the big toes touch each other. Keep the palms beside the thighs. While inhaling, raise the hands over the head and point the toes downward. Stretch the whole body, inhale and exhale slowly and deeply. While exhaling bring the hands down beside the thighs. Keep the eyes closed throughout the practice. Repeat this twice.

Benefits: A very good exercise for the lungs as it massages every air-sac and strengthens them. It is also useful in treating hypertension, heart disease, arthritis, bronchitis, back pain and shoulder pain.

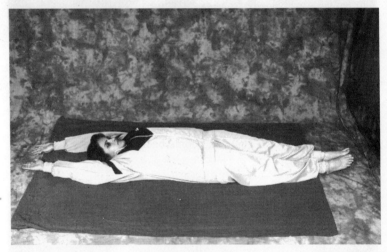

Uttan Tadasana

MERUDANDA SHITHILIKARAN (Relaxing Pose)

Lie on your back gently. Rest your legs on a chair. Gently close your eyes and try to relax the whole body mentally and physically.

Benefits: It is highly recommended in relieving stiffness of spine and back pain. Actually, it relaxes the whole spine and relieves tension.

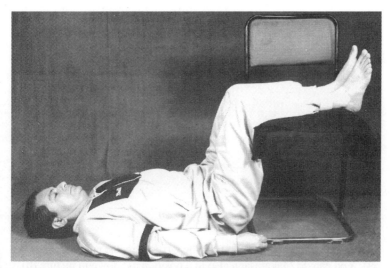

Merudanda Shithilkaran

PRONE POSES

MAKARASANA (Crocodile Pose)

Lie on your abdomen and cross your arms in such a way that the palm of one arm comes on the other shoulder. Keep your elbows down and spread

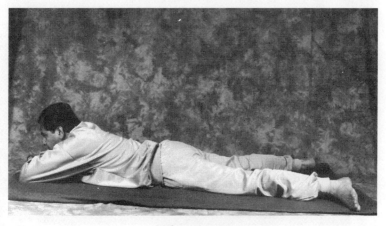

Makarasana (a)

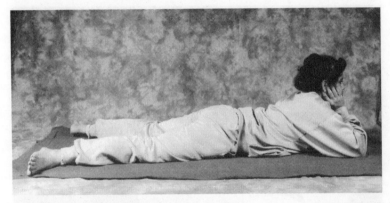

Makarasana (b)

them. Keep your chin between both the wrists. Breathe normally and take rest. You can do Makarasana also in a position as shown in picture (b).

Benefits: This is a simple and useful Asana to get relief from the tension of body and mind. The muscles get complete rest. This is very good in high blood pressure, heart disease and mental disorders. This also gives relief in back pain.

BHUJANGASANA (Cobra or Serpent Pose)

Lie in the prone position with the forehead resting on the floor, legs straight and feet together, toes pointing backwards, arms bent at the elbows, palms flat on the floor, shoulders and arms on the sides of the

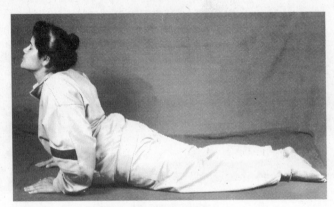

Bhujangasana

chest and fingers kept straight and together. Inhale and slowly raise the upper body (head, neck and chest). Look at the ceiling (sky) with the neck bent as far back as possible. For raising the body, only the back muscles are to be used. Do not push up with the arms. Waist, legs and toes should remain on the ground. Raise the body as much as possible. Hold the posture for a few seconds, breathe normally. Exhaling slowly, return to the original position. Repeat this twice.

Benefits: In diseases like cervical spondylitis, bronchitis, asthma and eosinophilia, it has a great therapeutic value. It removes weakness of the abdomen and tones up the reproductive system in women. It gives good exercise to the back muscles and vertebrae.

UGRA BHUJANGASANA

Lie down on your abdomen and relax in the Makarasana. Start the Asana by spreading both your hands and legs. While breathing lift your head, chest up to the navel and straighten your arms. Maintain this position for sometime. Inhaling and exhaling should be normal. Come back to the original position while exhaling. Repeat this.

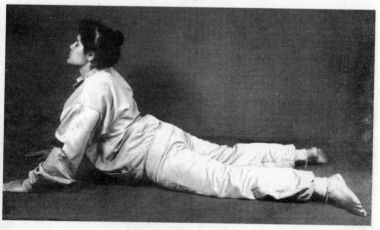

Ugra Bhujangasana

Benefits: It is beneficial in case of back pain.

SARPASANA

Lie down on your abdomen and relax in Makarasana. Start with taking both your arms at the back, make a finger lock with both your hands and put your

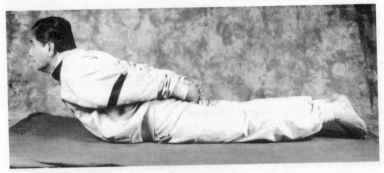

Sarpasanga

feet together. While inhaling lift your head and chest and stretch your
hands at the back. Maintain this position for some time and breathe
normally. Come back to the original position while exhaling. Repeat this
Asana twice.

Benefits: Useful in back and lower back pain. It also increases the
capability of inhaling and exhaling.

ARDHA SHALABHASANA (Half Locust Pose)

Lie down flat on the abdomen with soles of the feet facing upwards. Keep
both the hands under the thighs and rest the chin on the ground. Breathe in.
While raising the right leg without bending the knee, slowly and steadily
keeping the other leg and the trunk stationary, breathe normally. Now

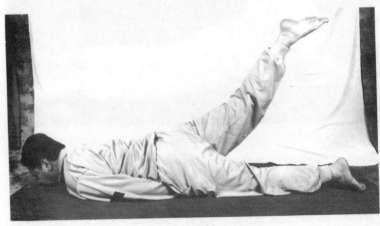

Ardha Shalabhasana

slowly lower the raised leg to the original position. Breathe out. Follow the same procedure for the left leg. Repeat the Asana twice on each side.

Benefits: It is one of the best exercises for the pelvis. By this any pain in the lumbar region, either due to wrong posture or pressure, could be relieved to a great extent. It also removes excess fat from the thighs, hips and abdomen. It helps to reduce protruding belly and makes the waist resilient and supple.

SHALABHASANA (Locust Pose)

Lie on the abdomen with legs stretched, and feet together, chin resting on the ground. Keep both the hands under the thighs. While inhaling, slowly lift both the legs upwards and stretch as far as possible without bending the knees and toes. Retain this position for some time and breathe normally then, while exhaling, lower the legs slowly and bring back to the original position. Repeat this twice.

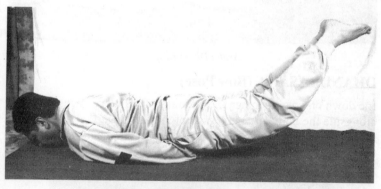

Shalabhasana

Warning: Persons suffering from hernia, cardiac complaints and ulcer should avoid this Asana.

Benefits: It is helpful in relieving arthritis and rheumatism. It strengthens the whole body, particularly the lungs, abdominal organs, sciatic nerves, prostate glands and the kidneys. It also gives relief in cases of diabetes, constipation, dyspepsia, bronchitis etc.

ARDHA DHANURASANA

Lie down with face and the forehead touching the ground, arms extended alongside the body and the legs straight. Now fold your right leg at the knee and hold it with the left hand and stretch your right hand forward. While inhaling, raise right leg and stretch the body to the maximum. Exhale back to normal. Repeat the same with other hand and leg.

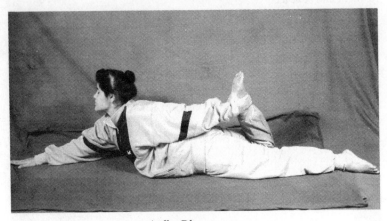

Ardha Dhanurasana

DHANURASANA (Bow Pose)

Lie down on your abdomen in Makarasana and relax. Arms extended alongside the body and the legs straight. Bend the legs at the knees towards the hips, bringing them forward so that they could be held firmly by the hands at the ankles on the respective sides. While inhaling, stretch

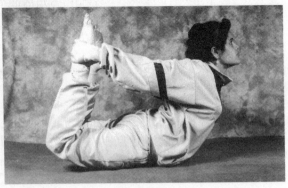

Dhanurasana

the legs backward and raise the thighs, chest and the head simultaneously. Hands should be kept straight. The weight of the body should be on the navel. Knees should be kept close, if possible look upwards. This posture should be retained, for at least a few seconds, breathe normally. While exhaling bring down the legs, hands and head to the ground. Repeat it.

Warning: This Asana should not be done by those suffering from a weak heart, high blood pressure, stomach and bowel ulcers and slipped disc.

Benefits: The abdomen, especially around the navel, and the chest muscles become strong. The throat, arms, shoulders, thighs, legs, lower back and abdomen, all become flexible. The spine also becomes healthy and strong. It is good for relieving flatulence, constipation and menstrual irregularities. It also prevents sterility.

NAUKASANA (Boat Pose)

Lie down straight on the abdomen with forehead resting on the floor. Keep the feet together and arms extended forward with palms on the floor. While inhaling, raise the arms, head, neck, shoulders, trunk and legs simultaneously as high as possible. Keep the elbows and knees straight. Balance the entire weight of the body on the navel. Maintain the posture as long as possible, breathe normally. While exhaling, bring down the legs, hands and forehead to the ground. Then relax in Makarasana.

Benefits: Naukasana improves the functioning of the lungs, useful in treating disturbed navel and relieves body stiffness and back pain. It also reduces excess fat from the abdomen, improves digestion and relieves constipation.

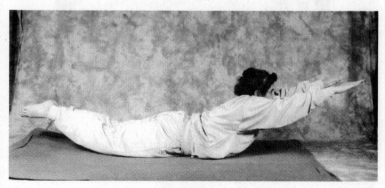

Naukasana

SITTING POSES

SUKHASANA (Easy Pose)

Sit on the floor with legs stretched in front. Fold the right leg at the knee and place it under the left thigh. Then bend the left leg and place it under the right thigh. Both the thighs should press the respective heels and to make it easier, adjust them without forcing the knee, feeling mentally and physically comfortable. Keep the head and the spine erect. Place the hands on the knees and close the eyes.

Benefits: Helps to calm the strained and irritable nervous system. Relieves muscular fatigue of the legs, knee and thigh joints.

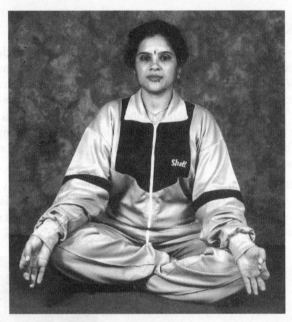

Sukhasana

ARDHA PADMASANA

Sit with legs stretched. Bend the right leg at the knee and hold the right big toe with the left hand and ankle with the right hand, gradually bring the leg towards the left thigh. Place the right foot as close as possible to the left thigh joint. Keep the left leg straight and slowly press the right knee on the ground and adjust the leg properly. Now fold the left leg also from the knee and bring it close to the right knee and place the left foot beneath the right thigh. Keep the spine, trunk and head straight. Place the hand on the knees and relax.

Benefits: Persons who find difficulty in performing Padmasana should practice this. This is a good posture for doing Pranayama and relaxation practices.

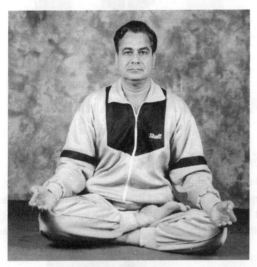

Ardha Padmasana

PADMASANA (Lotus Pose)

Sit on the ground stretching out both the legs in front. Bend the right leg at the knee and place the foot on the root of the left thigh. In the same manner fold the left leg and try to keep the left heel as close as possible to the root of the right thigh, so that both the heels touch each other as near the navel as possible. The head, neck and the spine should be kept straight and knees should touch the ground. Keep your hands in Chin or Jnana Mudra (see p. 103) and after some time slowly unfold the legs. The same can be repeated by changing the position of the legs.

Benefits: It strengthens and activates the function of the spinal nerves as those in the lower part of the spinal cord get good blood supply. It also helps in toning the inguinal parts and brings calmness and freshness to the mind.

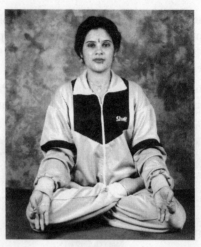

Padmasana

VAJRASANA (Pelvic Pose)

Sit comfortably, keeping both the legs stretched in front. Bend the right
leg at the knee and place the foot under the right hip. In the same manner,
fold the left leg and place the foot under the left hip. Try to adjust the feet
so that the toes touch each other and the heels are apart. Keep the knees

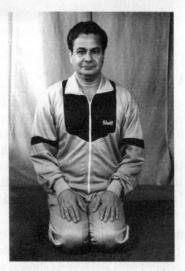

Vajrasana

together and let both the hips fit in between the heels. Place the hands on the thighs and keep the trunk and the neck erect.

Benefits: It improves the digestive capacity. Hence it could be done after meals.

JANUSIRASANA (Head Knee Pose)

Sit erect and stretch the legs forward. Bend the right legs so that its sole is against the left thigh. Press the perineum with the heel. While inhaling, raise both the hands over the head. Now exhale and bend forward and try to touch the left knee with the forehead. Hold the left toe with the right hand and let the left hand rest on the back. Right elbow should touch the ground, breathe normally. While inhaling, return to normal position. Repeat the procedure on the other side.

Warning: Those suffering from hernia, colitis and slipped disc should avoid this Asana.

Benefits: It helps to massage the heart and the abdominal organs. It is very useful in reducing excess fat in the abdomen, hips and thighs. It cures constipation, dyspepsia, seminal weakness, belching and digestive disturbances. It also helps overcome several menstrual disorders.

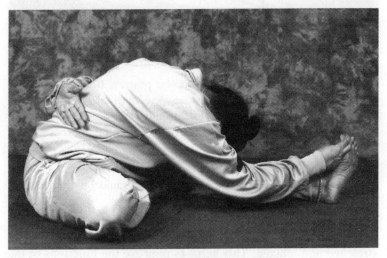

Janusirasana

PASCHIMOTTANASANA (Posterior Stretching Posture)

This posture involves stretching of the posterior muscles of the body. While sitting, stretch the legs forward and keep them close to each other. While inhaling raise both the hands over the head make hooks of the fingers and hold the big toes on the respective sides. While exhaling, bend forward stretching the trunk along the thighs. Make the face rest on the knees. Knees should be kept straight. Gradually, the tense muscles could

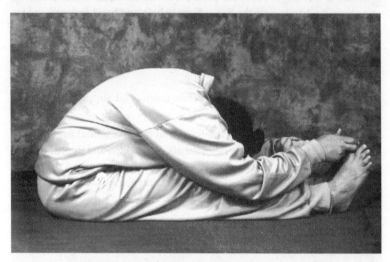

Paschimottanasana

be made supple for securing the complete posture. Breathe normally. Inhale and return to the original position. Aged persons and those whose spines are stiff, should do it slowly and steadily in the beginning. All jerky movements must be avoided. The stiffness can be overcome with patience and perseverance.

Warning: Persons suffering from slipped disc, hernia, lumbar spondylitis, cardiac problems and those who have undergone abdominal surgery should not perform this Asana.

Benefits: Paschimottanasana is a fine stretching exercise of the body. In one continuous movement, almost all the posterior muscles get fully stretched and relaxed. This helps to improve the functions of the abdominal organs and sets the respiratory disorders right. It also helps in improving memory.

USTRASANA (Camel Pose)

Sit between the heels and toes as in Vajrasana. Then raise the body upto the knees, laying the weight on the knees, keeping them slightly apart. Now raise the hands over the head and while inhaling, slowly bend backwards. Hold the right heel and then the left with the respective hand. While exhaling arch the spine and the neck fully. Push the pelvis forward. Retain the posture for sometime. Breathe normally and then return to the starting position.

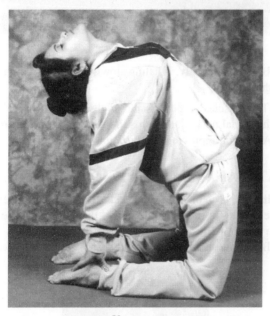

Ustrasana

Benefits: It tones up the abdominal viscera, particularly the liver, pancreas, kidney and bladder. It expands the chest and strengthens the ribs. It removes the sluggishness of the liver.

SASANKASANA (Hare Pose)

Sit with legs folded backwards, heels apart, knees and toes together. Adjust your hips between the heels (Vajrasana). While inhaling slowly, raise the arms over the head. While exhaling, slowly bend forward, stretch the palms on the floor with abdomen pressing against the thighs. Then bring the face downwards and touch the floor with the forehead without raising the

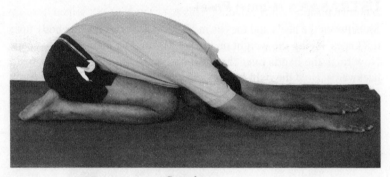

Sasankasana

buttocks. Breathe normally. Inhaling slowly, return to upright position, reversing the process.

Benefits: The muscles of the legs and thighs get stronger and supple. It tones up the spinal nerves and helps in relieving arthritic pain. It is an excellent Asana for improving the digestion.

PARVATASANA (Mountain Pose)

Sit in Sukhasana, keep the spine and neck straight. Close the eyes gently and inhale raising both the hands above the head. Join the palms in Namaskar Mudra. Elbows should be straight and hands stretched upwards. Breathing should be slow and deep. Feel the heartbeat. Return

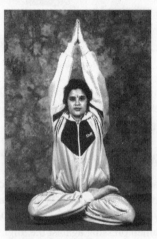

Parvatasama

to normal position while exhaling. This Asana may be performed three to four times.

Benefits: Parvatasana pulls up all the abdominal, pelvic and side muscles, stretches the spine and ribs. It gives natural massage to the heart and lung muscles. It is very useful in relieving the lumbar, spinal and shoulder pain and is good for hypertension also.

SKANDHASANA

Gently sit in Vajrasana or any other comfortable meditative pose. Place your hands on the shoulder and rotate both hands clockwise and anti-clockwise. Breathe normally.

Benefits: It relieves stiffness of shoulders, neck and back and strengthens the cranial nerves and shoulder muscles.

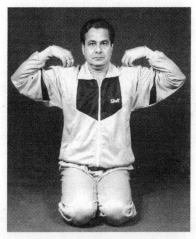

Skandhasana

HASTHA PARSHVASANA (Anchor Posture)

For Hastha Parshvasana, sit in any comfortable pose, entwine the finger of both the hands behind the back and while inhaling, stretch the chest forward and the hands backwards. At the same time, stretch the neck slightly backwards. While exhaling, come back to the normal sitting posture. Repeat this three to four times.

Benefits: It improves the functioning of the lungs, diaphragm, ribs and cardiac muscles. It helps in stooping shoulder.

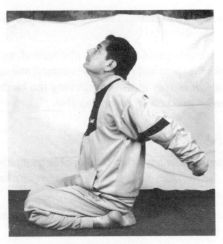

Hastha Parshvsana

VAKRASANA (Twisted Pose)

Keep the legs stretched in front. Raise the right leg by bending the knee
and pull the foot till it rests by the side of the left knee. Place the right
hand behind the back without much twist of the trunk. Then bring the left
arm over the right knee and hold the right ankle. Push the right knee as far
to the left as possible, offering good resistance to the left arm. Now exhale
and try to twist the trunk to the right side as much as possible, taking good
support from the left arm, and look towards the right shoulder. Breathe
normally. This is a complete twist to the right side. Do this Asana in the
same manner on the left side also. Do it twice.

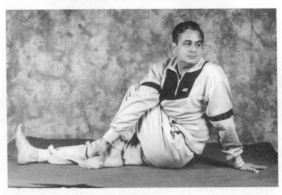

Vakrasana

Benefits: A very good exercise to make the spine flexible. It is helpful in treating enlarged and congested liver and inactive kidneys. Brings relief to hypertension, constipation and diabetic patients.

ARDHA MATSYENDRASANA (Spine Twist Pose)

Sit on the ground stretching both the legs forward. Bend the right leg and place the heel under the left hip. Now bend the left leg, cross it over and place the foot by the side of the right knee. Try to hold the left ankle by passing the right arm over the left side of the left knee. At the same time, exhale and take the left arm behind the back and press the right side under the ribs. This has to be done by twisting the trunk to the back as much as possible. Maintain this posture for a few seconds, breathe normally and increase the duration to two minutes gradually. Repeat the same process on the other side for the same duration.

Benefits: This exercises the spine and ensures its free movement. It also massages the liver, spleen, bladder, pancreas, intestine and other abdominal organs. This Asana stretches and strengthens the spinal nerves. It is highly recommended for treatment of obesity, dyspepsia, diabetes and urinary disorders.

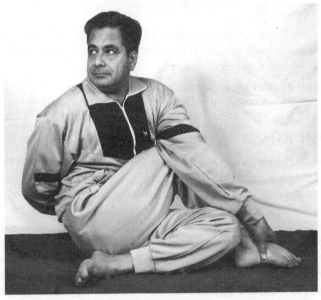

Ardha Matsyendrasana

66   *Yoga for Health*

MANDUKASANA (Frog Pose)

Take the posture of Vajrasana, fold your palms into fists and place them next to your navel. While exhaling, gradually bend forward without raising your hips and rest the abdomen and fists over the thighs. Retain the posture for some time breathe normally and while inhaling, return to the normal position and relax.

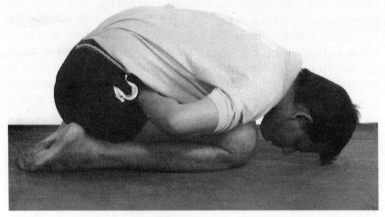

Mandukasana

Warning: People suffering from peptic or duodenal ulcer, severe back pain, cardiac problem and patients who have undergone abdominal surgery should avoid this exercise.

Benefits: Mandukasana improves functions of all organs. It is advised in the treatment of constipation, diabetes and digestive disorders.

GOMUKHASANA (Cow Face Pose)

Sit on the floor with legs out-stretched. Fold the left leg and bring the foot under the right hip. Similarly fold the right leg over the left and place the right heel by the side of the left hip. Both the soles should face upwards. Raise the right hand and bend it to bring it behind the shoulder. In the same way, bend the left hand behind the back and entwine the fingers and keep the spine straight. Breathing should be slow and deep. Note that if the right leg is over the left, the right elbow should face upward and left downward. This position may be reversed when the leg position is changed. Hold the posture for 30 seconds. Repeat the procedure reversing the sides.

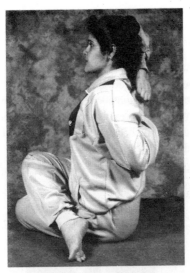

Gomukhasana

Benefits: Gomukhasana prevents enlargement of the testicles and calcium deposits on the shoulder joints. It is also helpful in treating sciatica and piles. It relieves muscular pain in the back and sprain in the forearms. It is one of the best Asanas for respiratory disorders, hypertension and cardiac complaints.

SIMHASANA (Lion Pose)

Sit on the heels with the knees apart. Keep your hands on the thighs in Chin Mudra with head downward as in Jalandhar Bandha. Mouth should be opened wide and tongue extended as far as possible towards the chin. Concentrate between the eyebrows. Breathing should be normal.

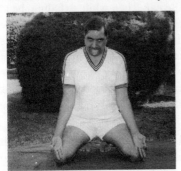

Maintain this posture as long as you can.

Benefits: Simhasana helps cure diseases of the face, tongue, vocal cords, back and anus. It removes nervous weakness and ensures longevity. It helps clear the voice and also improves the eyesight.

Simhasana

STANDING POSES

TADASANA

Stand straight and join your feet. Lock the fingers of both the hands and while inhaling, straighten them above your head. Stand on the tip of your toes. Looking straight will keep the balance automatically. Maintain this position for sometime and breathe normally. Come back to the original position while exhaling. Repeat this Asana.

Benefits: The stiffness of the body is relieved. It also gives relief in the neck, back and joint pain.

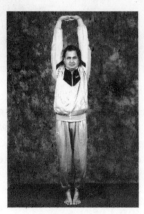

Tadasana

CHAKRASANA (In Standing Position)

Stand straight keeping your feet apart. Arms should be on the sides touching the body and hands should touch the thighs. While inhaling slowly, lift the right hand touching the ear. Then while exhaling, bend down as much as you can on the left side. Palm direction should be towards the floor. Try to keep your hand straight. This is the complete position of Chakrasana. Breathe normally and stay in this position for some time. Straighten your hand while inhaling. Come back to the original position while exhaling. Repeat this with the left arm too and this Asana is complete. You must feel that your body is bending towards one side. Repeat it twice.

Benefits: The spine becomes flexible and the back also stretched. It strengthens the liver, pancreas and kidney. With this rib muscles are also exercised. The hip-joint, lower back and shoulders also become flexible.

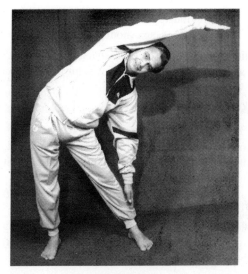

Chakrasana

KATICHAKRASANA

Stand straight keeping your legs apart. Now stretch your arm towards the shoulder's direction. Move the upper part of the body on the right side and bend your left hand while exhaling see at your back. Keep your right hand straight, maintain this position for some time. Breathe normally.

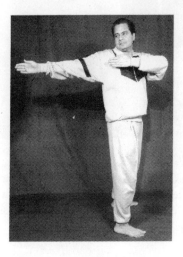

Katichakrasana

Come back to the previous position while inhaling. Repeat this on the reverse side. The complete Asana should be done twice.

Benefits: This Asana reduces the excessive fat from the waist and makes it flexible. It also massages the lungs. This helps in inhaling and exhaling.

NECK EXERCISE

Stretch your legs apart and keep your hands on your waist.
a)   Move your neck to and fro without giving a jerk. Do it thrice.
b)   After this move your neck from right to left and from left to right. Do it thrice.
c)   Now bend your neck from right to left and from left to right. Do it thrice.
d)   After this move your neck in a circular motion from right to left and left to right. While exercising breathing should be normal and eyes should be open. Do it thrice.

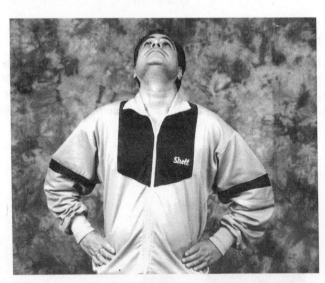

Neck Exercise (a)

Benefits: This is very good exercise for the neck and facial muscles. It helps remove the facial wrinkles and double chin. It massages the cranial nerve naturally. It benefits the most in case of insomnia. In vernal cranial (cervical) pain do not bend the head forward.

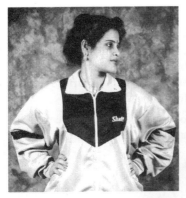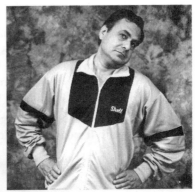

Neck Exercise (b & c)

SHOULDER EXERCISE

a) Join your feet and stand straight. Take a deep breath and while holding the breath close your feet and move your both the hands in circular motion at least five to six times and later bring them near to your chest and exhale while straightening them. Repeat it in the opposite order.

b) People who have pain in their shoulders, should keep both the hands on the shoulders (pic. b) and move them in circular motion first and then move in the opposite order. These can be done while sitting. *(Please see Skandasana.)*

Benefits: This exercise gives relief in pain in the back, neck, elbows, shoulders and joints of the upper part of the body.

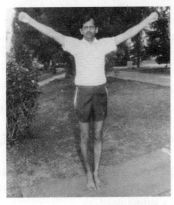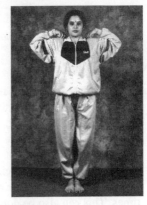

Shoulder Exercise (a & b)

ABDOMINAL EXERCISE

Stand with feet apart, slightly bend the legs at the knees and stoop forward. Place the hands on the knees. Now exhale fully and contract the abdomen towards the spine. Hold the breath and start pumping the empty stomach pumping till you feel comfortable. Then return to normal position and repeat the same three to four times.

Benefits: Abdominel exercise gives good exercise and massage to all the abdominal organs. It reduces the abdominal fat.

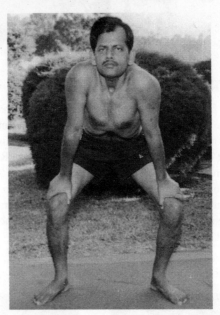

Abdominal Exercise

ANKLE EXERCISE

Stand erect with feet together, rest your palms on the waist.
1. Raise the right leg about six inches high. Move the ankle slowly up and down without jerking. Repeat it five times.
2. After this move the ankle from right to left and from left to right. Repeat it five times.
3. Now move the ankle in a circular motion from right to left and left to right. Breathing should be normal during the exercise. Repeat it five times. This can also be done in a sitting position.

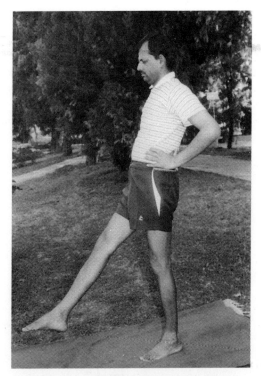

Ankle Exercise

Benefits: This exercise gives relief in the ankle pain and also develops the muscles and ankles remain in a good condition. One can practice it while sitting also.

KNEE EXERCISE

1. Sit on a chair or on a hard bed. Slowly swing both the feet to and fro.
2. Put the heel of the right foot on the toes of left foot and move it up and down ten to fifteen times. Similarly do with the left foot also.
3. Hold your right thigh with both the hands and straighten it and later bring it slightly towards the chest and press it with both the hands. Do it ten to fifteen times. Similarly do the exercise with your left thigh.
4. Sit on a hard bed and straighten your foot. Move it a little up and down. It massages the knee-cap.

5. Stand erect, keep both the palms on the thighs. Then bend at the knees, keeping the back straight. The knees can be moved to the left and right also.

Benefits: This is a good exercise for removing stiffness and pain in the knees as in arthritis.

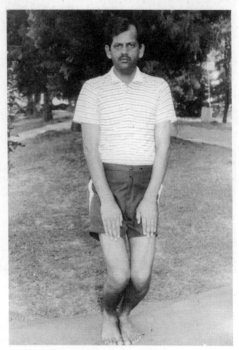

Knee Exercise

SHIRSHASANA (Topsy-turvy Posture)

Kneel down and make a finger lock by inter-locking fingers of both the hands. Place the finger lock on the seat in front of you, keeping the elbows apart and place the forehead on the floor supported by finger lock. Start raising the feet so that the calf muscles touch the thighs. Breathe normally. This is the first stage and should be maintained perfectly, because the balance during the final posture depends mainly on this stage.

In the next stage, raise the knees first and then slowly raise the feet so that the complete body is straight like a pillar. This is the final stage. Breathe normally. Come back to the original position by reversing the process.

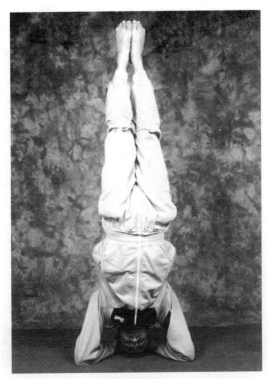

Shirshasana

SHIRSHASANA (On Apparatus)

This is much easier, comfortable, safer and better than doing it directly on the floor without any support. Place the apparatus near the wall. Then conveniently place the shoulders on the pads of the stand. Support the body by gripping the sides of the apparatus and gradually lift the body straight up. If necessary, support the legs against the wall. Breathing should be normal. Balance the whole body on the apparatus. While returning to original position, slowly bend the knees and gradually bring the leg down to the floor. After Shirshasana, relax in Shavasana.

Caution: Avoid jerky movements at all stages. Maintenance of balance comes by continuous practice. For securing proper balance, elbows are to be placed firmly on the ground in the same line as the finger lock. While performing Shirshasana on the apparatus, shoulders should balance properly on the pads. In the beginning this Asana should be done only for

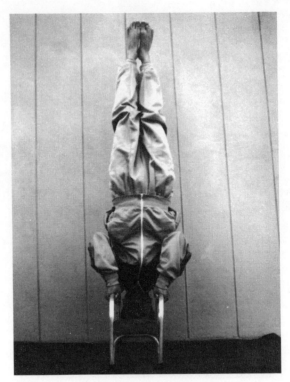

Shirshasana (On Apparatus)

10 seconds with the help of someone. Then the time could be increased gradually by half-a-minute every week.

Warning: Those suffering from discharge from the ears, iritis, high blood pressure, heart problems, severe cervical and lumbar spondylitis should not practice this Asana. It should be practised under the guidance of an expert.

Benefits: Improves the blood supply to the brain and working efficiency of the nervous system. Endocrine glands also become healthier as they get good blood supply. This Asana is helpful in cases of dyspepsia and constipation. It improves the functions of the reproductive glands and heart muscles and is of great advantage in checking wet dreams.

VI

EYE CARE

Yoga therapy has a role in the treatment of myopia and other refractive errors beside general improvement of eyesight and general health. Yogic exercises of extra ocular muscles help to strengthen and relieve the strain or tension upon these muscles to overcome the defective vision.

The following eye exercises are advocated for better eyesight.

1. **Sun Treatment:** Early in the morning, look at the rising sun. Gaze the sun till the rays emerge. Avoid looking at the emerging or hot sun.
2. **Swing:** Stand straight comfortably with feet apart, facing the sun. Keep the hands relaxed. Gently close the eyes and sway the whole body from one side to the other.

   The sun is the source of energy which tones up and increases the working efficiency of all the six eye muscles and increases the blood circulation to the eye.
3. **Splashing:** After the sun treatment, go under a shed. Fill the mouth with cold water. Cup your palms, fill with cold water and splash over the eyes. Do the same at least seven to eight times and gently wipe later.
4. **Blinking:** Sit straight comfortably. Make short and rapid movements of the eyelids, i.e. close and open the eyelids rapidly. Repeat three to four times followed by palming.
5. **Gazing at the Thumb:** Sit straight in any comfortable posture. Stretch both the arms forward upto the shoulder level. Raise the thumb upward and fold all the fingers. Now move the left thumb to the left side till it is in line with the shoulders and follow the movement with the eyes without moving the neck and head. Then bring it back and repeat with the other hand. Then do the same upwards and downwards. Keep the right hand above the shoulder and left hand on left thigh. Gaze at the thumb up and down and sideways. Repeat on the other side by changing the hands and lastly

move clockwise and anti-clockwise. After that rub the palms together and place them over the eyes gently. Eyes must remain closed for some time. The body should be motionless during the practice.

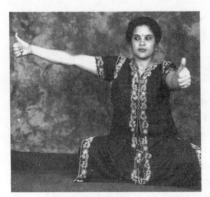
Eye Exercise - A

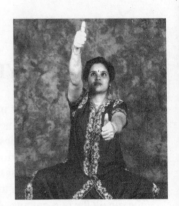
Eye Exercise - B

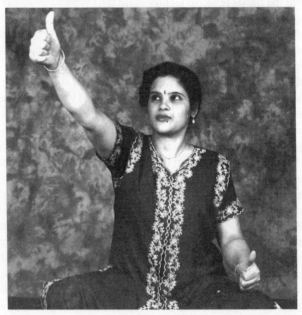
Eye Exercise - C

6. **Bhrumadhya Dristi (Frontal Gaze):** In this Kriya, the eyesight has to be fixed between the eyebrows. It is good for checking the wandering nature of the mind. It also removes dullness and lethargy.

7. **Nasikagra Drishti (Nasal Gaze):** The eyesight has to be fixed at the tip of the nose without winking. It may be practised in any of the meditative postures like Siddhasana, Sukhasana, Padmasana or Vajrasana.

This Kriya increases stability and concentration of the mind, strengthens the optic nerves, corrects weakness and certain eye disorders. It cures insomnia if practised at night before sleep.

8. **Gazing at the ball:** It is done by playing with a ball from one hand to the other. Or, throw a ball to the ground and observe the bounces. One should follow the ball's movements. The ball playing exercise improves the accommodation ability of the eyes. Do it three to four times.

9. **Trataka:** Trataka is an eye exercise which is done by concentrating on a pre-decided object.

    Sit at ease in dhayana posture. Head, neck and back should be relaxed. Keep one lighted candle or a lamp one metre away from the eye. Close your eyes. Sit calm and relaxed and feel the body. After this open your eyes in a normal way, look and concentrate on the

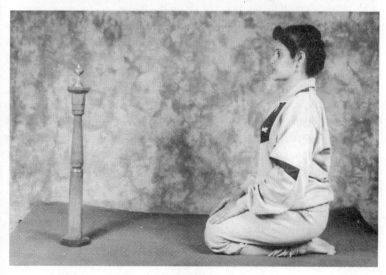

Trataka

flame of that candle or a lamp without winking your eyes. At this time you see everything which is in the light of the flame that is why focusing is required here. With this gradually you stop seeing things surrounding the light, only the flame is visible. This second step is called fixing. Reaching to the last position, i.e. merging, where subject and object merge and become one, is difficult but reaching the second stage is also beneficial for improving the eyesight and the will-power which helps in living your life.

Precaution: During this if your eyes feel exhausted or there is some irritation, stop the exercise immediately. Close your eyes, relax for some time and then start again. If eyes become watery, continue the exercise. The patients having eyesight problem should consult their doctor before starting this.

How many times: This can be done at any time but doing it early morning or late night for 15 to 20 minutes is much better.

Important Points

1.   This Kriya should be done under the guidance of an expert.
2.   One should not move during the entire exercise.
3.   One should not wink or rotate the eyes during the exercise.
4.   In case of a burning lamp or a candle, it should be done in a closed room so that the air does not affect the flame.
10. **Steam Inhalation:** 30 seconds to 1 minute, steam inhalation by adding a few eucalyptus leaves. Place your head in the facial (steam) sauna, gently close the eyes. After that, splash cold water and wipe it gently.
11. **Palming:** Sit comfortably, close the eyes gently and rub your palms. Cover them with the palms in such a way as avoiding any pressure on the eyeballs and without allowing the light to pass through. If it is not completely dark before the eyes during palming, and some other colour appears, it indicates that the eyes and mind are under strain. This may be practised for minimum 2 to 3 minutes.

Note: After Trataka and Facial Steam (Vapour) relax in Shavasana.

Benefits: This is one of the best exercises for removing tension, fatigue and myopia. Regular practice improves eyesight. It is a very good exercise for the eye muscles and the optic nerves.

VII

BREATHING AND RESPIRATION

Though in common usage and both the terms mean the same, respiration has a wider meaning. Breathing is a physical or mechanical act in which oxygen from the air enters the body and then the air along with impurities such as carbon dioxide and water vapour are expelled.

Respiration, on the other hand, includes the act of breathing, as well as the process of carrying the absorbed oxygen to every part of the body. Oxygen is indispensable for life. The important aspect of carrying oxygen to each minute part of the body is done by the blood. Breathing may be called as internal respiration, as it helps in the supply of oxygen internally.

Though in Pranayama the breathing activity is controlled by bringing into action impulses from the brain, *prana* (breath) and *chitta* (mind) are in fact inseparable. They are interdependent. Ancient masters of Yoga knew that the mind can be controlled by controlling the breath through Pranayama.

Breathing can be controlled voluntarily to a certain extent. The average rate of respiration of an individual varies from 16 to 20 breaths per minute. All the air we breathe in, does not reach the alveoli. A part of it is retained in the nose, trachea and bronchi. They also contain exhaled air which is again breathed in. This is called dead space. In quiet breathing, the quantity of fresh air that enters the lungs is about 5 litres per minute. This is known as the minute volume.

The respiratory centre has two parts – namely, the inspiratory centre and the expiratory centre. The inspiratory centre has motor nerves and sensory nerves which connect it to the diaphragm and the external intercostal muscles along with the wall of alveoli. The expiratory centre is also closely connected with the internal intercostal muscles and the muscles of the abdomen. When the nerves are stimulated respectively, the muscles contract causing inspiration and expiration.

Pranayama provides systematic massage to the abdominal muscles and also tones up the working of spleen, liver, kidney, pancreas, intestines and adrenal glands. Puraka, Kumbhaka and Rechaka should be practised in symetrical proportion and increased systematically. If one inhales for 8 seconds, retention and exhalation should be for the same length of time, which works out to a ratio of 1:1:1. This should be gradually increased to 1:1:2 and later to 1:2:4. Pranayama improves the efficiency of respiratory, circulatory and nervous systems. Deep breathing increases intake of the oxygenated blood which in turn increases the red blood corpuscles. Pranayama, in particular, strengthens the nervous system (*Nadi Mandala*), *Ida*, *Pingala* and *Sushmana*, which are situated at the base of *Nadi Mandala*. It has more than 72,000 *Nadis*. *Nadi* does not mean nerve. *Ida*, situated in the left nostril, also known as Moon *Nadi*, gives a cooling effect to the system. *Pingala* flows through the right nostril, known as Sun *nadi*, gives internal warmth (heat) to the body.

Sushmana, situated in the spinal column, flows for a brief period during the day and the night. This is related to the spiritual aspects of life.

When both the nostrils are dominating, that is the time to meditate and concentrate the mind on a particular subject. When the right nostril is active (breathing faster) vigorous practice of Hatha Yoga, hard work, taking a bath, exchanging news of any serious matter, sleeping or sexual contact can be done. When *Pingala* is dominating the system, it produces more chemical changes by improving internal heat. It also produces more gastric juice which helps in digestion. When the left nostril is dominating, it is time to meditate, visit holy places, enjoy music – bhajans, kirtans and dance. These three *nadis* are responsible for physical, mental and spiritual state of a human being. Pranayama, practised with Kriyas and Asanas under the guidance of Yoga expert, can cure many of the disorders like maladjustment of the personality, irregularities connected with menstruation and uterus, gout, arthritis, spondylitis, insomnia, sciatica, nervous problems, asthma, common cold, hypertension, piles, acidity, dyspepsia, flatulence, constipation, obesity, diabetes, backache and migraine including postural defects.

PRACTICE OF COMPLETE BREATH

The practice of complete breath makes a person immune to many ailments, particularly cold, bronchial diseases and other general weaknesses. Deep breathing allows the lungs to remain active and helps in resisting the germs that invade the lung tissues. The oxygenated blood nourishes the entire system.

The stomach along with other digestive organs is nourished by oxygen obtained from deep breathing. The food is absorbed by oxygen before it is digested and assimilated. Improper breathing results in reduction in body vigour, loss of appetite and impairment of the nervous system. It makes the minute nerves ineffective in transmitting nerve impulses.

DIAPHRAGMATIC RESPIRATION

The diaphragm is a membrane which separates the lungs and thoracic cavity from the abdominal organs. When one inhales deeply, the diaphragm expands (lower down) and helps to absorb the maximum quantity of oxygen. While exhaling, the diaphragm relaxes and rises, forcing the lungs to expel carbon dioxide.

To perform diaphragmatic or abdominal breathing, lie flat on the back, keeping the legs together and arms at the sides, with the entire body relaxed. Then inhale slowly and deeply, simultaneously making the abdominal muscles move outwards to the maximum extent. Hold the breath for a while. Then exhale slowly and deeply, allowing the abdominal muscles to move inwards to the maximum extent. Concentrate on abdominal movements only, without moving the chest.

Benefits: Correct diaphragmatic respiration gives effective movement to the abdominal organ and offers a natural massage to the cardiac muscles. It also improves the functioning of liver, pancreas, spleen, kidney, stomach and intestines.

CHEST BREATHING

The chest houses the lungs, which are protected by the ribs. During respiration, the ribs and the upper portion of the chest move, particularly during the inhalation. Due to this the chest cavity and the lungs expand bringing in much oxygen. While exhaling, it relaxes and removes carbon dioxide. During this period, an exchange of gases take place, thus purifying the blood.

For performing chest breathing exercises, lie down flat on the back, keeping the legs together and arms on the sides. Then inhale slowly and deeply, moving the chest cage and the ribs upward. While exhaling, the ribs will move downwards. This exercise will strengthen the trachea, thoracic region and air-sacs.

LUNG-BREATHING EXERCISES

A. Sit in any comfortable posture and stretch both the hands in front and close the eyes. While slowly inhaling, count from one to four and raise both the hands above the head and then hold the breath for two counts. While exhaling, count one to six and bring down the arms to

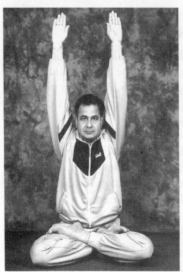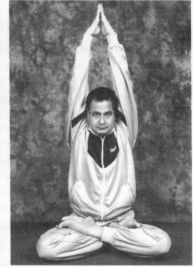

Lung-Breathing Exercise (a & b)

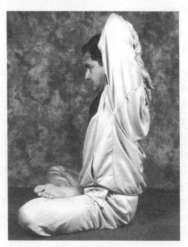

Lung-Breathing Exercise (c)

the original position, and then hold the breath for two counts. Repeat the exercise four to six times.

B. Sit straight and keep the hands above the head in Namaskara Mudra. Elbows should be straight and the eyes closed. Now inhale for four counts, then hold the breath for two counts. Exhale for six counts and again hold the breath for two counts. This may be practised four to six times.

C. Sit straight, keeping both the hands behind the shoulders and palms in the opposite directions. Try to keep the elbows straight upward and as far as possible, together with the chin a little low, and eyes closed. Inhale for four counts. Then hold the breath for two counts. Exhale for six counts, holding the breath for two counts. This exercise should be repeated four to six times.

Benefits: All the three lung-breathing exercises help opening up the tree-like section of the lungs, absorbing sufficient amount of *prana* (oxygen). They improve the lung capacity and provide natural massage to each and every air-sac in the lungs. They clean the entire respiratory system making the respiration smooth and easy.

VIII

PRANAYAMA

As per Yoga scriptures, Pranayama is the gateway to the deeper relaxation and meditation and is a scientific method of controlling the breath. It is practised to control the body and the mind. It makes one steady and peaceful for achieving the pure consciousness stage (samadhi).

The science of Yoga discovered the existence of *prana* and mastered the techniques to control it. In Sanskrit, "prana" has many meanings. It is equated to breath, respiration, life-force, cosmic energy, air, power, strength or the master control of all that lives, which pervades the entire cosmos. *Ayama* signifies length, abstinence, regulation, control and restraint. Thus Pranayama is the act of control of breath and an attempt to control the physical manifestation of *prana* in the human body.

It is also a regulation of breathing to integrate vital forces. Life and breath always go hand in hand, and they totally depend on each other. Hatha Yoga makes use of Pranayama techniques to derive many benefits for our physical and external existence.

Patanjali said that by practising Pranayama, one develops the power of concentration and clarity of thought. It helps in increasing the mental and physical powers of endurance.

Ayurveda says the entire system of the body is governed by three *doshas*, viz, *vata* (wind), *pitta* (bile) and *kapha* (mucus). The field of action of the three *doshas* is mainly between the navel area and the heart. This area is most vital in the human body, where the oesophagus, diaphragm, cardiac sphincter, stomach, duodenum, liver, pancreas, spleen, kidney, ileum, caecum and colon are located. This area is also responsible for digestion, assimilation and distribution of nourishment. Even a slight imbalance in them creates disturbance in the whole system.

Vata controls the action and movement in the human system, *pitta* the whole digestive system and *kapha* moistens and lubricates the joints which keeps the body clean and neat. They are present all over the body. *Pitta* and *kapha* are classified into five kinds based on their nature and location in the body.

WHAT IS PRANA?

The *vayu* or *vata* (wind) keeps the system alive and its nature changes with the variation in the temperature. Of the three *doshas*, *vayu* is the most important. By controlling *prana*, one can control all the forces of the universe, viz, gravity, magnetism, electricity and nerve currents. Thus *prana* refers to the energy as the basis of all life and is traditionally divided into five main forces, known as Pancha Prana.

Ancient Indian sages knew that the functions of the body were performed by five types of vital energies. They are Prana, Apana, Samana, Udana and Vyana with separate manifestations and distinct functions.

Prana functions in the thoracic region. It is known as the life breath which activates respiration and operates in the heart and the lungs. Prana, also known as nasal breathing, is located between the larynx and the upper part of the diaphragm, including the chest and maintains the life system by filtering and warming up the air taken in through the nose.

Apana circulates in the lower abdomen, between the navel and rectum, including the large intestine and the reproductive organs. It expels the waste materials from the system and helps in the elimination of urine and faeces. It is also responsible for bleeding, labour pain, child birth, abdomen ache and the semen.

Samana circulates between the heart and the navel centre, including the small intestine and the umbilical region. It stimulates the gastric fire, activates and controls the digestive system and maintains the harmonious function of the digestion separating nutrients from waste. The main function of the Samana is to maintain the balance between Prana and Apana.

Udana circulates in the throat region, located above the pharynx, larynx, nose and tongue. Udana is responsible for the sore throat, sinus, headache, earache and speech problems like stuttering (stammering).

Vyana circulates along the whole body distributing the energy from the food and breath, through the lymphatic and nervous system. Actually, Vyana controls the body systems, including the flow of blood, elimination of toxins and coordination of every body activity.

Like this Prana also consists of five Uappranas, as Naga, Kurma, Krikal, Devadatta and Dhananjay. Naga Prana is responsible for belching, hiccuping, Kurma Parana Devdutt is winking the eyes, Krikal Prana for thirst, hunger and sneezing, Devdutt Prana for yawning and Dhananjay Prana is responsible for destroying the last cell of the dead body completely.

Another vital aspect of scientific and therapeutically aspect of Yoga is Pranayama. Pranayama is the breathing process or the control of the motion of inhalation, exhalation and the retention of vital energy.

During Pranayama, Puraka (inhalation) stimulates the system, enlarges the chest cavity and fills the lungs with fresh air. Kumbhaka (retention) which increases the carbon dioxide level in the blood, raises the internal temperature and plays an important role in increasing the absorption of the oxygen. During Rechaka (exhalation), the diaphragm returns to its original position and air full of toxins, and impurity is forced out by the contraction of the intercoastal muscles. These are the main activities during the Pranayama which gives systematic massage to the abdominal muscles and also tones up working of spleen, liver, kidney, pancreas, intestine and adrenal glands. Due to proper function of these organs, vital energy flows to all the systems. The proper ratio should be maintained among Puraka, Kumbhaka and Rechaka. The ratio should be increased gradually. Scientific breathing helps in proper expansion and relaxation of the respiratory apparatus. Deep breathing technique helps in proper supply of oxygen to the system. It helps in elimination of unwanted gas from the stomach and intestine, generate *prana*, brings smoothness in the nervous system and also gives natural massage to the alveolar air-sacs.

Pranayama also provides complete relaxation to the nervous system. The expansion of lungs during deep breathing, moves ribs, intercoastal muscles and even the vertebrae, thus providing relief from pain caused due to compression of nerve ending.

Pranayama should be practised in a place full of fresh air, free from dust, insects and bad odour. Avoid all sorts of disturbing factors. Ideal time is the early morning when the mind is fresh and the atmosphere cool.

During Pranayama, bandhas like Jalandhar, Moola and Uddiyan play a very important role in maintaining the flow of *pranic* energy to the particular areas. Above mentioned bandhas are fully responsible for maintaining the body activity by proper utilisation of oxygen. It reduces the rate of respiration thereby increasing the lifespan. Pranayama helps in increasing oxygen supply to the brain which in turn helps control the mind.

AANA PAAN

Aana Paan and Sukha Pranayama are very good for relaxing the body and mind. It gives strength to the nerves and the breathing system. Sit in any of the meditative posture and relax. Head, neck and spine should be erect. Rest your palms in Chin or Jnana Mudra on your knees. Close your eyes. Concentrate on your natural breathing system and feel how breath is coming in and out of your lungs. Breathing should be normal. Minutely inspecting the inhaling and exhaling is Aana Paan.

SUKHA PRANAYAMA

Sukha Pranayama provides deep relaxation to the mind and the body, improves concentration and strengthens the nervous and the respiratory systems. It is useful in relieving depression, anxiety, hypertension, lack of concentration and cardiac problems.

Sit comfortably in any meditative posture with head, neck and spine straight. Keep the palms on the knees and assume Jnana or Chin Mudra. Close the eyes. Then observe your natural breathing and feel the touch of breath on the tip of the nose. Slowly feel the flow of breath in and out of the lungs. Let the breathing be natural and automatic. Do not change the rhythm of breathing. Feel and observe the abdominal movement.

Just inhale and exhale very slowly and rhythmically. While inhaling, let the abdominal wall slightly move out and while exhaling, let it go in. Keep the chest immobile. While doing this, feel that with every inhalation you are drawing in cosmic energy, vital power and peace, and with every exhalation you are throwing out tension, disease and impurities. Have a clear mind and do not entertain any other thought in your mind.

KAPALBHATI

Kapala in Sanskrit means skull and *bhati* is to shine or to clean. It cleanses the respiratory tract, including the nasal passages and the capillaries of the lung. It helps in the elimination of gases from the lung and purifies the frontal portion of the brain. It aids in combating chronic bronchitis, asthma, cerebral thrombosis, diabetes and nervous disorders caused by excessive wind, bile and phlegm. It relaxes and revitalises the mind by improving concentration. Though the Yoga text has not mentioned Kapalbhati as one of the Pranayamas, it has remained as one of the six Kriyas – purification or cleansing techniques of Yoga.

A.   To perform Kapalbhati, sit comfortably in any comfortable posture, preferably in Padmasana, with spine, neck and head erect. Rest your hands on the respective knees and be relaxed. Exhale through both the nostrils, contracting the middle and lower portions of the abdomen. Release the contraction of the abdominal muscles quickly and follow at once with another forceful expulsion of breath. Increase the frequency, finally to reach 120 strokes per minute. After completing the rounds take a deep breath and exhale slowly.

B.   Sit straight in a comfortable meditative posture. Place the left hand on the left knee. Exhale through alternative nostril actively and forcefully by adopting Nasikagra Mudra on right hand (as shown in the picture).

The important points to be observed during the Kapalbhati are:

1.   The chest and the shoulders should be kept immobile during the entire practice.
2.   Exhalation should be vigorous, accompanied by the contraction of abdomen, whereas inhalation should be effortless and passive.
3.   Neither should there be any pause between two strokes nor any retention of breath.
4.   The exhalation should be uniform in force and rapidity and the rhythm should be maintained.

Warning: Persons suffering from lumbago, high blood pressure and serious cardiac and respiratory disorders should practice Kapalbhati very slowly under expert guidance.

BHASTRIKA

As explained in *Hathayoga Pradipika,* Bhastrika Pranayama may be practised in various ways. Bhastrika in Sanskrit means bellows. It consists of forceful and quick inhalation and exhalation. The sound produced due to this resembles that of the bellows of a blacksmith.

A.   Sit straight in any comfortable meditative posture with head, spine and neck erect. The mouth should be closed. Left hand should be kept on the left knee in Chin or Jnana Mudra and right hand in Nasagra Mudra. (Index and the middle fingers should touch the palm.) Press slightly the right thumb on the right nostril and close it tightly. Now exhale through the left nostril and immediately inhale through the same actively and forcefully. Then quickly open the right nostril, by closing the left, exhale through the right. Immediately inhale through the right and quickly exhale through the left by closing the right nostril. Repeat it quickly.

During the practice of Bhastrika and Kapalbhati, the facial muscles should be relaxed. Keep the shoulder and the chest immobile, but relaxed. They should be performed as per one's capacity and strength. During these exercises if you sweat, do not wipe it with a towel, but rub the body with the palms.

B. Sit straight in a comfortable meditative posture. Place both the hands on the knees. Exhale and inhale through both the nostrils actively and forcefully.

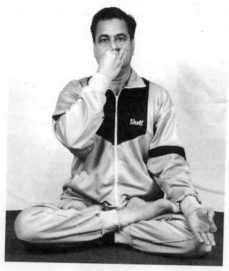

Bhastrika

Warning: Those suffering from hypertension, ischaemic heart disease, ulcers, vertigo and severe backache should abstain from doing these exercises. However, in some cases, it may be practised under the guidance of a Yoga expert.

Benefits: Bhastrika Pranayama is good as it strengthens the whole respiratory system, including bronchial tubes and the diaphragm. It will help to hold the breath longer. As air is forcefully drawn in and out, phlegm is removed by force. This purifies the blood stream and improves the working of the nervous system. Bhastrika helps improve the functions of the digestive organs, the sinuses, stops running nose and gives relief to bronchitis and asthma patients. It also maintains the body temperature and metabolic rate. It helps in reducing excess fat in the abdominal region.

SURYABHEDANA

In Suryabhedana Pranayama, the Surya Nadi – the right nostril is used for inhalation and the left for exhalation and hence the name Suryabhedana. Surya is the sun, which maintains the lungs and health-producing heat in the body. In Suryabhedana, inhalation is done through the right nostril and exhalation through the left nostril.

Sit in a meditative posture – Padmasana, Sidhasana or Vajrasana – keeping the neck, head and back straight. Place the left hand on the left knee in Chin or Jnana Mudra. Keep the left nostril closed with the ring and last fingers of the right hand. Without making any sound, slowly inhale as much air as possible through the right nostril. Close the right nostril with the thumb and exhale very slowly, without making any sound, through the left nostril by closing the right one. Advanced practitioners should maintain the ratio of the inhalation, retention and exhalation at 1:4:2 like in Anuloma-Viloma Pranayama.

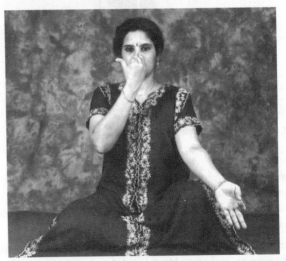

Suryabhedana

Benefits: Suryabhedana increases the body temperature by activating sympathetic nerves. It is one of the best Pranayamas for a running nose, cold, cough, bronchial asthma, diabetes and constipation. It purifies the brain cells and makes them healthy. It helps in relieving gastric fire, indigestion and destroys the internal worms. It promotes catabolic activity of the body which helps to reduce weight.

CHANDRABHEDANA

In Chandrabhedana Pranayama, the left nostril (*chandra nadi*) is used for inhaling and right nostril for exhaling and that is the reason this Pranayama is called Chandrabhedana.

Sit either in Padmasana or in Vajrasana. Keep your neck, head and back erect. Keep your left hand in Chin Mudra on your left knee. Make Nasikagra Mudra with your right hand, close your right nostril with your right thumb and inhale through the left nostril slowly. Then close the left nostril and exhale through the right nostril. Then immediately close it and again inhale from the left and exhale through the right nostril. Repeat this.

Benefits: Chandrabhedana Pranayama helps in increasing anabolic activity to increase the weight if done on an empty stomach, 27 times four times a day. It helps in maintaining the peace within and to lower down high blood pressure by activating parasympathetic nerves. It also promotes coldness in body.

Note: Start all the Pranayamas exhaling from the left nostril.

ANULOMA-VILOMA

There are varieties of Pranayama. They differ with regard to Puraka and Rechaka and the inhalation and exhalation rate. In Kumbhaka, the retention part of *prana* is the most effective part and it is also practised in various degrees, depending on the *sadakas*.

A. Sit straight in Padmasana or in any meditative posture. Keep your left hand on the left knee in Chin or Jnana Mudra. Make Nasikagra Mudra with the right hand and close the right nostril with your thumb. Now slowly exhale through the left nostril and then very slowly inhale through the same with the right nostril still closed. Retain the breath by closing the left nostril. Then open the right nostril and exhale slowly through it. Again inhale through the right nostril slowly, close it and retain the breath. Then open the left nostril and slowly exhale. This completes one round of simple Anuloma-Viloma. Retention of breath should not be more than one's capacity.

B. Assume any comfortable Asana. Place the left hand on the left knee in Chin or Jnana Mudra and close the right nostril with your right thumb. Slowly exhale through the left nostril and then inhale very slowly through the same. Now close both the nostrils and tuck your chin into your throat cavity. This is Jalandhar Bandha.

After sometime, release Jalandhar Bandha and slowly exhale through the right nostril at double the length of time taken for inhalation. Again slowly inhale through the right nostril, close both the nostrils and lock into Jalandhar Bandha. After a while release Jalandhar Bandha, slowly exhale through the left nostril as before. This completes one cycle of Pranayama. Maintain the ratio 1:2:2, i.e. if you are inhaling (Puraka) for a count of four, retention (Kumbhaka) should be for eight counts and exhalation (Rechaka) eight counts. Gradually the retention count may be increased.

C. Sit erect in Padmasana or any comfortable meditative posture. Keep the left hand on the left knee in Chin or Jnana Mudra and the right thumb on the right side of the nose, fourth and fifth fingers on the left side of the

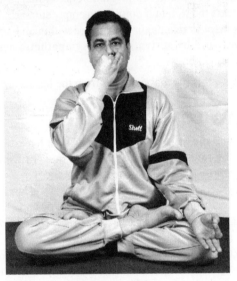

Anuloma-Viloma

nose. Fold the index and middle fingers. Do not twist the nose. Only slightly press the bony region to control breathing. Now slowly exhale through the left nostril and inhale through the same. Close both the nostrils and perform Jalandhar Bandha. Simultaneously contract the anal region and perineum in Moola Bandha and retain the breath according to your capacity. Then release Jalandhar Bandha and Moola Bandha and slowly exhale through the right nostril with double the time taken for inhalation. While exhaling, contract your abdomen to perform Uddiyana Bandha, keeping the left nostril closed and maintain the rhythm while exhaling. Repeat the same process with the right nostril.

This completes one cycle of Anuloma-Viloma. Gradually increase the time, the ratio of inhalation, retention and exhalation of the breath upto 1:4:2 During the practice, inhaling and exhaling should be done very slowly without any sound. After completing the round, come back to normal position. Continue for 3 to 4 minutes. Close the eyes and feel the vibrations of Anuloma-Viloma Pranayama.

Benefits

1. Anuloma-Viloma Pranayama includes two each of the three components. A round consisting of all the procedure, profoundly enriches the supply and flow of *prana*. It maintains the body temperature and metabolic rate, purifies the blood stream, the nervous system, the brain cells and increases the serenity of the mind. It maintains flexibility of the arteries, veins and capillaries and prevents ischaemic heart disease and improves general stamina and vitality of the body.

2. It is also mentioned that during breathing, cells receive nutrition, strengthening the nerves and endocrine system. The flow of pure blood to the entire body is maintained by contraction of diaphragm by involving the concerned rhythmic use of abdominal muscles and parts of respiratory system. In Anuloma-Viloma, one has to inhale through one nostril, retain the breath, then exhale through the other nostril.

3. Anuloma-Viloma improves the working of the respiratory system and increases the lungs' capacity for oxygen intake. It maintains the flexibility of arteries, veins and capillaries. It also controls the cholesterol and sugar levels in the blood and improves the working efficiency of thyroid and parathyroid glands, liver, pancreas and kidney.

It helps in controlling asthma, diabetes, constipation and insomnia. Patients suffering from hypertension and cardiac problems must refrain from holding the breath in Anuloma-Viloma.

Puraka (inhalation) will stimulate the system, enlarge the chest cavity, fill the lungs with air and move the diaphragm down. Kumbhaka (retention), which increases the carbon dioxide level in the blood increases the temperature and the absorption of oxygen and tones up the tissues. During Rechaka (exhalation), the diaphragm returns to its normal position and air loaded with toxins and other impurities is forced out due to the contraction of the intercostal muscles.

UJJAYI

Hathayoga Pradipika says Ujjayi means producing sound loudly by a partial closure of the glotties, along with retention of the breath. There are two types of Ujjayi Pranayama.

Inhalation and exhalation by partially closing the glotties produces a frictional sound called Ujjayi. Sit erect in any comfortable meditative posture. Keep your hands in Chin Mudra. Now inhale slowly and deeply through both the nostrils with a low, uniform frictional sound through the glottis and expand the chest naturally. Then exhale through both the nostrils, taking double the time of inhalation giving the same frictional sound. Relax the chest simultaneously in a natural way. Complete the required number of rounds. Advanced practitioners can fold the tongue inside in Khechari Mudra (see p.104).

Benefits: Ujjayi Pranayama helps in relieving allergic cold, swelling of tonsils, removal of phlegm from the throat and improves lung capacity. It is useful in treating hypertension and insomnia. It tones up the nervous system and improves the oxygen supply. It calms the mind and helps maintaining good health.

SHEETALI, SHEETAKARI AND SADANTA – COOLING PRANAYAMA

Sheetakari, Sadanta and Sheetali Pranayama involves breathing through the mouth, which refreshes the person and quenches thirst. Sheetakari Pranayama helps in controlling thirst, hunger and sleep. It also improves the digestion and purifies the blood.

SHEETALI

Sheetali cools the nervous system, improves the working of the liver, spleen and the digestive system, purifies the blood and removes toxins from the system. It is also very useful in treating fever, high blood pressure and mental tensions.

In Sheetali Pranayama, one should inhale the air through the mouth, specially through the tongue muscles which produces a cooling effect on the system. Therefore, it is called Sheetali.

To perform Sheetali, sit erect in any comfortable posture, keeping both the palms on the knees in Chin or Jnana Mudra. Close the eyes. Draw out the tongue about one inch from the lips. Roll it up from the sides to form a tube, like a bird's beak. Then slowly and deeply suck the air

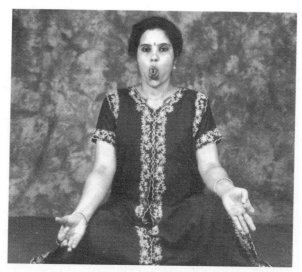

Sheetali

through it and fill the lungs completely. After full inhalation, withdraw
the tongue and close the mouth.

Retain the breath inside for a while and slowly exhale through both
the nostrils. Complete the required number of rounds. Depending upon
the condition of the patient. It is advisable not to practice it in the winter
months.

SHEETAKARI

Inhalation is through the mouth rather than the nose in Sheetakari
Pranayama. One has to produce a hissing sound, while sucking air over
the tongue and that is why it is called 'Sheetakari'.

Sit erect in a comfortable position. Keep your hands in Chin Mudra.
Slightly open the mouth keeping the lips open. Then slightly press the tip
of the tongue in between the teeth and then suck the air slowly through the
mouth with a 's-s' hissing sound. After sucking the air completely in,
close the mouth and slowly exhale through both the nostrils. Sheetakari
may be performed with the bandhas. Complete the required number of
rounds.

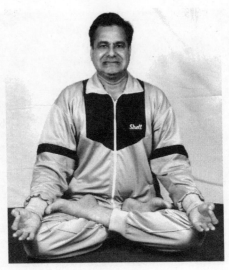

Sheetakari

SADANTA

Sit in a relaxed posture. Keep your hands in a Chin Mudra. Slightly open your mouth and tighten your teeth and inhale through the gap of the teeth and close your mouth and exhale through the nose. This helps to bring the bacteria out of the teeth thus cleans teeth and on the other hand it cools the body.

Benefits: Sadanta Pranayama helps to treat the disease like pyorrhoea. Regular exercise activates the salivary glands which helps in digestion. A special benefit is that it prevents the bad mouth odour.

BHRAMARI

Bhramari Pranayama promotes a sweet, clear voice and is highly recommended for singers. It is also useful in preventing insomnia, tension, depression, hypertension and nervous disorders. It is very beneficial for women during pregnancy in preparation of labour. Bhramari is also known as humming breath, as the sound produced during exhaling resembles the humming of a large bee and hence the name 'Bhramari'.

Sit erect in any comfortable meditative posture. Relax the body completely. Inhale slowly and deeply through both the nostrils. Inhalation

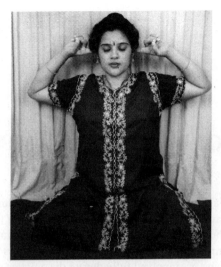

Bhramari

should be clear, vibrating the throat area and giving a very soothing effect to the whole nervous system. Then gently plug the ears with the corresponding index fingers and close the eyes. While exhaling, produce a long and continuous humming sound like that of a bee.

Benefits

The sound and vibrations produced during Bhramari are absorbing and soothing. It makes an impact on the mind producing peace and joy. During Bhramari Pranayama, blood circulation increases in the brain hence memory power increases. This is also known as 'laya' Pranayama because it gives lulling affect to the brain. Thus very useful in insomnia.

IX

ROLE OF BANDHAS AND MUDRAS

Technically Jalandhara Bandha, Moola Bandha and Uddiyana Bandha are the three main bandhas, which are performed during the practice of Pranayama. These bandhas stimulate Mooladhara, Manipuraka and Vishudha *chakras* and control mental state. These *chakras* are situated in the spinal cord and get involved fully during the practice of Pranayama. They play a role in maintaining the *pranic* energy in a particular area by holding, pressing, lifting and pulling, while performing a physical action. Bandhas also give a massage to the endocrine and nervous systems, improving *Ida, Pingala* and *Sushmana nadis*. These three *nadis* are mainly responsible for maintaining oxygen balance in the system.

JALANDHAR BANDHA (Chin Lock)

Jala in Sanskrit means net. Sit in any meditative pose with palms on the knees, the neck and the spine straight. Relax the whole body. Then inhale slowly and deeply through the nose, lifting the chest naturally and stretching slightly the cervical area. Fix the chin tightly in the jugular notch. Retain the breath as long as possible. Then release the lock and the neck while exhaling.

Before starting the next round, take a few normal breaths. During the performance of Jalandhar Bandha, the air is completely sealed in the thoracic region and the effect that produces through physiological action, on the lungs is like that of a net.

Jalandhar Bandha which is directly related to Vishudha Chakra, which is responsible for storing the energy in the form of *prana*, strengthens the *Sushmana Nadi* and ensures harmonious balance between the endocrine glands and the respiratory system. Jalandhar Bandha monitors the working of the Medulla Oblangata, which is situated above

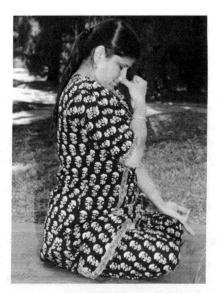

Jalandhar Bandha

the spinal cord and the pituitary gland, the master gland. It also gives positive vibrations to particular arteries and capillaries supplying blood. While improving the voice of the person, it gives a natural massage to the thyroid and parathyroid glands in the throat.

MOOLA BANDHA (Anal Contraction)

Contraction and release of the anal region and the perineum is Moola Bandha. To perform Moola Bandha sit in Siddhasana or Padmasana with the knees touching the ground to make it easy for applying pressure on the perineum. It can also be performed in any Asana, but the above two Asanas are ideal. Keep the palms on the knees and slightly press them. Gently close the eyes and relax, both mentally and physically.

Now, inhale slowly and deeply through the nostrils and perform Jalandhar Bandha (tuck the chin into the throat cavity). Then contract the muscle between the anus and the genitals, including the pelvic region and the perineum, and lift upwards. Be in this posture holding the breath as long as possible. Then release the pressure on the anus and other related organs, simultaneously releasing Jalandhar Bandha. Exhale slowly.

Before performing Moola Bandha, it is advisable to practice Ashwini Mudra by contracting and releasing the anal muscles several times with proper breathing. This would help practice Moola Bandha in a proper manner.

Moola Bandha stimulates the Mooladhara Chakra and maintains the balance between Prana and Apana Vayu and improves the working efficiency of the sympathetic nerves.

Moola Bandha is directly related to Pranayama. The practice of Moola Bandha along with Pranayama and Jalandhar Bandha, controls the flow of *prana* and maintains the energy of the body. It stimulates and activates the nervous and respiratory system and helps to eliminate toxins from the body. It improves digestion, relieves gas and painful menstruation. It strengthens the adrenal glands, intestines, reproductive organs and Mooladhar Chakra.

UDDIYANA BANDHA (Raising the Diaphragm)

Raising the *prana* from the lower abdomen to the brain and to contract, restrain or tie it, is called 'Uddiyana Bandha'. It is basically an exercise of the diaphragm, ribs and the lower abdomen, which may be done in a sitting or standing position. During Pranayama, Uddiyana Bandha is to be practised only in the sitting position.

Sit in any meditative posture relaxing the entire body and close the eyes. Inhale deeply and then exhale fully securing the deepest possible expiration. Immediately perform Jalandhar and Moola bandhas by tucking the chin into the throat cavity and contracting the anal region upwards. Press the hands on the knees, (with empty lungs), so that the neck and shoulder muscles are in a fixed position. Then pull back the

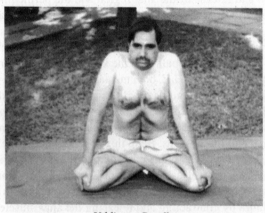

Uddiyana Bandha

entire abdominal region towards the spine by lifting the diaphragm up and creating a concave shape of the abdomen. Hold the breath as long as possible. Then relax the abdomen. Release the Jalandhar and Moola Bandhas allowing the abdomen to return to the normal position. Before starting a new round, breathe normally for some time. It should be performed only on an empty stomach.

Uddiyana Bandha stimulates the Manipuraka Chakra, which is situated just behind the navel centre. This is a zone of energy and as per Yoga philosophy, the navel is the centre of energy. During Uddiyana Bandha, diaphragm and abdominal muscles move vigorously up and down as well as backwards. As a result cardiac muscles, respiratory organs, liver, spleen, adrenals, pancreas, kidneys and intestines get toned up and their functioning improved by the elimination of toxins from the body. This Bandha is helpful in treating constipation and diabetes.

ROLE OF MUDRAS

Bandhas and mudras are fundamentally related to each other and they play a crucial role together during the performance of Pranayama and Asanas. Mudras bring the senses under control and help in concentrating one's mind on a single point like the Pratyahara, the fifth step of Astanga Yoga, which is also the gateway to Antaranga Yoga (Internal Yoga)

Mudra are the precursors to Pratyahara, in which the *sadhaka* could secure perfect control over the *indriyas* (senses). Mudra means gesture, regarded as stimulate. They tone up and control the nervous system. They also control the *pranic* energy and involuntary physiological function by giving a smooth pressure on a particular point. In Yoga texts more than 25 types of mudras are mentioned.

Chin Mudra

Sit erect. Fold the index finger and touch on the first joint of the thumb. Let the other three fingers be spreaded and relaxed. Keep the palms on the knees facing upwards. Chin Mudra gives a soothing effect to related nerves, improving concentration.

Jnana Mudra

Sit erect. Join the tips of the index fingers and thumbs. Let the other three fingers spread. Then place the hands on the knees facing downwards and close the eyes. Maintain natural breathing. Jnana Mudra activates *vayu* and improves vital energy. It helps in controlling the mind and reducing the rate of respiration. It helps in increasing grasping power.

Khechari Mudra

Sit erect in any comfortable meditative pose. Fold the tongue and let its tip go back into the throat as far as possible to the nasal cavity. The tongue may push the upper palate of the mouth. Khechari Mudra, in advanced stages of practice, requires expert guidance. It improves the efficiency of the vital organs, salivary glands, pituitary and pineal glands and helps to improve memory by giving a soothing effect to the brain cells.

Ashwini Mudra

Sit straight relaxing the whole body. Keep the palms on the knees. While inhaling, contract the anus and while exhaling release the anal muscles. Ashwini Mudra is a preventive exercise for piles, prolapsed of the uterus, rectum and prostate. It is helpful in cases of constipation and gastritis.

Yoga Mudra

Can be done in any meditative posture, including Vajrasana, but Padmasana is more beneficial. Sit in Padmasana keeping the spine straight. Inhale deeply and grasp the wrists behind the back and exhale slowly. Then bend the trunk forward keeping the hands at the back.

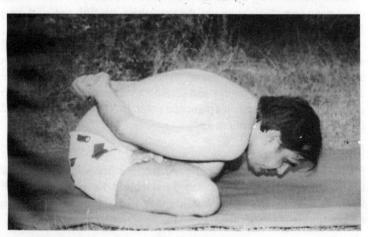

Yoga Mudra

Gradually bring the face down, the head touching the floor. Retain the posture as well as the breath as far as possible. Relax the neck and cervical region.

Inhale, slowly return to the upright position in the reverse order. The extra pressure on the abdominal muscles improves the peristaltic movement of the intestines, strengthens the prostate glands and reproductive organs. Yoga Mudra also helps in improving digestion.

It relieves constipation and balances the vital energy between Vishuddha and Mooladhara Chakras.

Maha Mudra

Sit erect. Stretch the legs together forward. Bend the right leg and place the heel under the perenium. While exhaling bend forward and hold the left big toe with the hands by keeping the leg straight. Then inhale slowly and deeply and simultaneously perform Moola Bandha keeping the head and spine straight. Retain the breath inside as long as possible and then exhale slowly. Repeat the same by changing the position of the leg. Maha Mudra gives a natural massage to the cardiac muscle. It helps in prostate and seminal weakness.

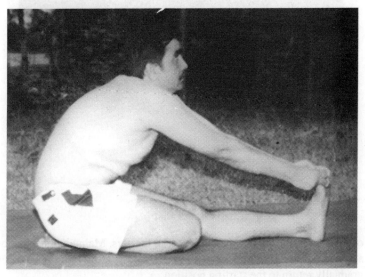

Maha Mudra

Tadagi Mudra

A. Sit straight and stretch the legs forward fully as in Paschimottan-asana. Keep your legs slightly apart. Then bend forward and hold the big toes by the respective hands. Inhale slowly and deeply and let the abdominal wall expand fully. Retain the breath for some time. During this period relax the whole body and exhale slowly. Still remaining in the same position, pump the abdomen with inhalation and exhalation. Then finally release the posture with exhalation.

B.   Lie down in Shavasana. Raise your knees and bring the feet nearer to
the hips. Keep the hands near the thighs. Now inhale and raise the
abdomen fully. Then exhale fully, hold the breath outside and
contract the abdomen. Now pump your abdomen vigorously. Do it
six to eight times and then relax.

Pashini Mudra

Lie flat on the back with the legs and feet together, arms beside the thighs.
While inhaling, raise both the legs together pushing them above and
behind the head so as to touch the floor. Bend the legs at the knees and
bring them towards the face. Keep the knees close to the ears and
shoulders as in Karnapeedasana. Hold the wrists tightly around the back

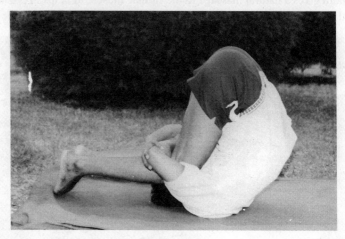

Pashini Mudra

of the legs and try to bring them closer to the ears. Maintain this position
as long as possible and keep the respiration slow and deep. Then
gradually return to the starting position.

Pashini Mudra stimulates and tones up the Medualla Oblangata, the
nervous system and the vertebral column. It reduces excess fat of the
abdomen, controls diabetes and improves the working efficiency of liver,
spleen, kidney and intestines.

Vipareeta Karni Mudra

Lie flat on the floor with arms straight and close to the body, palms facing
downward. While inhaling raise the legs together and place the palms on

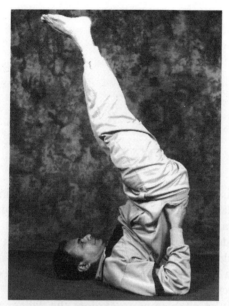

Vipareeta Karni Mudra

the waist, balancing the body on the shoulder blades and the hands. The chest should not press against the chin. Now inhale deeply and expand the abdominal muscles and while exhaling, relax the abdomen. This is a way to gentle abdominal breathing. While exhaling, gradually return to the original position bringing the legs down slowly.

Vipareeta Karni Mudra improves the blood circulation in the abdomen, chest, neck and brain, tones up the lungs, cardiac muscles, kidneys, liver, spleen and the inner surface of the stomach.

X

YOGA NIDRA

Everything else in life may deceive you, but the determination made on Yoga Nidra can never go waste. Once a resolution is made with the help of Yoga Nidra, your mind will always stand by you.

Yoga Nidra is a powerful technique for relaxation. It is a systematic method of inducing complete physical, mental and emotional relaxation. During Yoga Nidra, one appears to be asleep, but the consciousness would be functioning at a deeper level of awareness.

Yoga Nidra enables us to explore the deeper realms of the subconscious mind, thereby releasing and relaxing the mental tensions and establishing harmony in all respects.

Recently, diseases with new dimensions have appeared. Among them a few are stress-related disorders caused by our inability to adapt to the highly competitive pace of a modern life. The real problem for these diseases lies not in the body but in man's changing ideals, lifestyles, thoughts and feelings. These maladjustments lead to tension and hypertension and many other psychosomatic diseases.

Psychosomatic illnesses such as diabetes, hypertension, migraine, asthma, ulcers, digestive disorders and skin diseases arise because of tension. Cancer and heart diseases too arise from tension. If one knows how to control tension, one could easily control anger, passions and emotions and their resultant diseases such as heart ailments, high blood pleasure, leukemia and angina pectoris.

Yoga Nidra is a more efficient and effective form of psychic and physiological rest and more rejuvenating than conventional sleep. In fact, a single hour of Yoga Nidra is equivalent to four hours of conventional sleep.

Yoga Nidra is a state of mind between wakefulness and sleep. It opens the deeper phase of the mind, the subconscious mind. This subconscious mind is very obedient and disciplined and immediately carries out the orders it receives. By practising Yoga Nidra, the subconscious mind could be completely trained. The ordinary or the conscious level of the mind and intellect would follow suit.

HOW TO PRACTISE YOGA NIDRA

First of all lie down in Shavasana. If you want to cover yourself with a *chadar* (cotton sheet) you can. Close your eyes while arranging your cloths and body. Relax and let loose if any part of the body is stressed. Listen to the instructions carefully. Do not engage yourself in any thought or plan and keep your mind free from all thoughts. Be careful that you do not move your hands and legs during this practice. Lie down in a position as you do before going to sleep but do not sleep. Just listen and concentrate on the instructions.

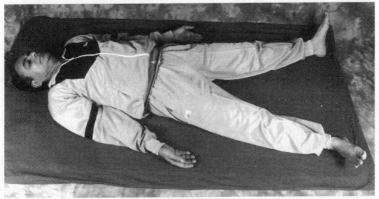

Yoga Nidra

If you practice Yoga Nidra with all your heart, you will attain eternal bliss. Now we will try to understand what is Yoga Nidra. It is an effective and systemic way of bringing the relaxation mentally, physically and emotionally. The person in Yoga Nidra seems to be asleep but his conscious is active somewhere deeply in his body. Yoga Nidra keeps you away from the mental tension. Yoga Nidra is an effective and a good way of relaxing psychologically and physically both. One gets more relaxation by Yoga Nidra than the normal sleep. In fact, one hour's Yoga Nidra is equal to hours of normal sleep.

Now you make a commitment... a commitment that is done with a feeling of complete surrender and faith towards God or make a commitment to stay healthy till the last moment of life or say that, "I am going to practise Yoga Nidra." Repeat your commitment thrice within yourself. Now see the things with closed eyes inside the Yoga-classroom, the roof of the room where you are lying, things around you... like wall, pictures on a wall, windows, carpet on which you are lying... and carefully see your body from head to toe... feel it. Now focus your consciousness on one part of the body.

Now feel the forehead and head... right eye... left eye... right eyebrow... left eyebrow... and the centre of both eyebrows carefully. Your right ear..., left ear... right check... left check... nose... both nostrils... upper lip... lower lip... chin... and go through all these parts mentally.

Look at your right hand... thumb of the right hand... second finger... third finger... fourth and fifth... tips of the fingers, palm... wrist... elbow... shoulder... right chest... right back... right thigh... knee... calf muscle... ankle... toe and lower side of the right foot... thumb of the right foot... and feel the rest of fingers.

Now look at your left hand... thumb of the left hand... second finger... third finger... fourth and fifth finger... tip of the fingers... palm... wrist... elbow... shoulder..., left chest, left back... left thigh... knee... calf muscle... ankle... toe and lower side of the left foot... thumb of the left foot... and feel rest of the fingers.

Now concentrate on your back... right shoulder... left shoulder... spine and each and every vertebrae of the spine from top to bottom... now concentrate your thought on the main parts... full right foot... left foot... feel both feet together... now feel full right hand... full left hand... and feel both the hands together... your full back and spine... like this full abdomen... chest... and the whole face... feel them mentally... your face is totally cool, stable and peaceful... now feel your whole head and body together... your body is lying on the floor completely stable and relaxed.

Now feel the normal breath... you are inhaling and exhaling. Beware that the breath is coming and going. Feel that you are inhaling from the right nostril and then from the left or sometimes from both, is our breath deep and long or short, is it warm, or cold, where it is touching that we have to experience, recognise and besides minute supervision of the inhaling and exhaling. Now concentrate on your abdomen – with every breath it is coming up or going down. Feel, while inhaling the abdomen comes out and exhaling it goes inside. Inhaling the breath, coming out abdomen exhaling the breath and sucking the abdomen inside should be done together and experience it.

Remember the moments of joy, happiness, and the bliss you experienced in your life. In this happiness, experience the early morning… Imagine and feel in this pleasant morning you are strolling at the banks of river… the continuous transparent water of the river with a gurgling sound is covering from the sky high mountains… The river is flowing with a clean water. Cool air is embracing the river. Cool air is also embracing you and you are enjoying it. In this peaceful atmosphere your heart is going deep in the peaceful sea. You are feeling that on the both sides of the river there are green fields all over, the birds are singing – in such a morning you are taking a stroll by the riverside – the sun is rising behind the mountains – whose rays are spready in the horizon.

The soft rays of the sun are absorbing in each and every cell and the energy is continuously spreading in the body. While walking you are entering a riverside temple, sitting in the front of a shivalinga you are surrendering with complete faith and belief to the One who is the Creator and Preserver. Only God's dhyana and worship… Each and every moment you are experiencing the happiness and bliss which is on the cosmic and inner level. And now you again repeating your commitment that you repeated three times that you will remain healthy till the last days of your life. Return to your body…

Now concentrate on your breath inhaling and exhaling. When you inhale the abdomen comes out and when you exhale the abdomen goes inside. Now start back counting from twenty-seven to one… like when your abdomen comes out and goes inside your count twenty-seven… and again your abdomen comes out and goes inside twenty-six… again when it comes out or goes inside twenty-five… Count upto one in the same manner. Count with concentration up to one (Pause for a minute).

Now stop counting and move your hands and legs slowly, but do not open your eyes. Turn to your right side and slowly get up and sit… Now rubs both your palms and keep on your eyes… Now slowly open your eyes. This is the end of Yoga Nidra.

REMEMBER

- Yoga Nidra is not at all a method of concentration, but a definite key for opening all the closed doors of your personality.
- On returning from work, immediately practise Yoga Nidra for five to ten minutes. It helps to relax.

- Yoga Nidra should be practised on an empty stomach. Do Yoga
  Nidra at least 3 hours after meals and ½ hour after light refreshments
  as the production of digestive enzymes are greatly reduced during
  Yoga Nidra.

The most important is, not to fall asleep during Yoga Nidra. If you feel
sleepy before doing it, take a cold shower.

XI

YOGA CARE FOR DISEASES

Yogic Management and Curative Value of Yogic Kriyas, Asanas, Pranayama and relaxation technique for various diseases. Also consult an expert in Yoga therapy.

1. **Amoebiasis and constipation**
   - Kriyas (K)- Kunjal.
   - Asanas (A)- Matsyasana,
     Pavan Muktasana,
     Tadagi Mudra,
     Bhujangasana,
     Shalabhasana,
     Janusirasana,
     Shavasana.
   - Pranayama (P)- Kapalbhati,
     Bhastrika,
     Anuloma-Viloma.

2. **Indigestion, loss of appetite and gastro-intestinal diseases**
   - K- Kunjal.
   - A- Pavan Muktasana,
     Tadagi Mudra,
     Bhujangasana,
     Shalabhasana,
     Yoga Mudra, Vakrasana.
   - P- Kapalbhati,
     Bhastrika,
     Anuloma-Viloma.

3. **Tension, stress, irritability, depression, anxiety, insomnia and sleeplessness**
   - K- Sutraneti,
     Jalaneti,
     Kunjal (salt-free),
     Eye Tonic.

	A-	Shavasana, Sarvangasana, Matsyasana, Dhanurasana, Janusirasana, Shashankasana, Shirshasana.
	P-	Kapalbhati, Anuloma-Viloma, Sheetakari, Yoga Nidra.
4. Liver disorder (Hepatitis) and amoebic liver	A-	Vipareet Karni, Matsyasana, Vakrasana, Tadagi Mudra, Pashini-Mudra, Shashankasana, Uddiyan Bandha.
	P-	Bhastrika, Suryabhedana, Anuloma-Viloma, Yoga Nidra.
5. Asthma	K-	Vastra Dhauti, Kunjal, Sutraneti, Jalaneti, Steam inhalation, Laghu Shankha Prakashalana (LSP).
	A-	Suryanamaskar, Bhujangasana, Dhanurasana, Paschimottanasana, Ustrasana, Shashankasana, Gomukhasana.
	P-	Bhastrika, Suryabhedana, Anuloma-Viloma, Yoga Nidra. Sutraneti.

**6. Bronchitis, allergic-
rhinitis, sinusitis, oesinophilia**

K- Kunjal, Steam inhalation, Jalaneti, LSP.

A- Suryanamaskar,
Sarvangasana,
Matsyasana,
Pavan Muktasana,
Ustrasana,
Bhujangasana,
Shalabhasana,
Dhanurasana.

P- Kapalbhati, Bhastrika,
Anuloma-Viloma.

7. Headache, migraine

K- Kunjal, Jalaneti, LSP.

A- Suryanamaskar,
Vipreet Karni,
Pavan Muktasana,
Bhujangasana,
Shalabhasana,
Parvatasana, Vakrasana,
Shavasana.

P- Sukhapranayama, Kapal-
bhati, Sheetali,
Sheetakari, Bhramari,
Yoga Nidra.

8. Hypertension (HBP)

A- Ardha Halasana,
Ardh Pavan Muktasana,
Uttan Tadasana,
Katichalana,
Parvatasana,
Vakrasana,
Shavasana.

P- Sukha Paranayama,
Lung-Breathing,
Anuloma-Viloma,
Sheetali, Sheetakari,
Bhramari, Yoga Nidra.

116

9. **Nervous debility, anaemia, underweight, hypotension (LBP)**

K- Kunjal.
A- Ardha Halasana,
Ardha Pavan-
Muktasana,
Uttan Tadasana,
Katichalana,
Parvatasana,
Vakrasana.
P- Bhastrika,
Anuloma-Viloma,
Bhramari,
Yoga Nidra.

10. **Diabetes Mellitus**

K- Kunjal, LSP.
A- Suryanamaskar,
Dhanurasana,
Pavan Muktasana,
Janusirasana,
Ardha Matsyendrasana,
Ustrasana,
Shavasana.
P- Kapalbhati, Bhastrika,
Suryabhedana,
Anuloma-Viloma,
Bhramari.

11. **Arthritis, rheumatism (Mobile)**

A- Ardha Pavan Muktasana,
Skandhasana,
Katichalana,
Uttan Tadasana,
Bhujangasana,
Shalabhasana,
Vakrasana.
P- Lung-Breathing,
exercises, Kapalbhati,
Bhastrika,
Anuloma-Viloma.

12. **Cervical and lumbar spondylosis**

A- Ardha Halasana, Ardha-
Pavan Muktasana (simple),
Katichalana,

		Setubandhasana, Bhujangasana, Ardha-Shalabhasana, Vakrasana, Parvatasana, Shavasana.
	P-	Lung-breathing exercises, Anuloma-Viloma, Bhramari, Yoga Nidra.
13. Kidney diseases	K-	Kunjal (salt-free).
	A-	Pavan Muktasana, Bhujangasana, Shalabhasana, Dhanurasana, Vakrasana, Shavasana, Uddiyan Bandh, Moolabandha.
	P-	Kapalbhati, Bhastrika, Anuloma-Viloma, Bhramari.
14. Gastric and duodenal ulcer	A-	Ardha Halasana, Uttan Tadasana, Ardha Pavan Muktasana, Parvatasana, Shavasana.
	P-	Sukha Pranayama, Sheetali, Anuloma-Viloma, Bhramari, Yoga Nidra.
15. Colitis	K-	Kunjal (salt-free).
	A-	Pavan Muktasana, Bhujangasana, Shalabhasana, Vakrasana, Padmasana, Shavasana, Moolabandha.
	P-	Lung-breathing exercises, Sheetali, Bhramari, Yoga Nidra.

16. Enlargement of prostate gland   K-   Kunjal, LSP.
                                        A-   Suryanamaskara,
                                             Pavan Muktasana,
                                             Sarvangasana,
                                             Matsyasana,
                                             Bhujangasana,
                                             Shalabhasana,
                                             Gomukhasana,
                                             Vajrasana,
                                             Yoga Nidra,
                                             Moola Bandha,
                                             Ashwini Mudra.

                                        P-   Kapalbhati,
                                             Anuloma-Viloma.

17. Skin diseases   K-   Kunjal (salt free).
                                        A-   Suryanamaskara,
                                             Dhanurasana,
                                             Paschimottasana,
                                             Ustrasana, Supta-
                                             Vajrasana, Shirshasana.

                                        P-   Anuloma-Viloma.

18. Hyper acidity   K-   Kunjal (salt free), LSP
                                             (with less rock salt).
                                        A-   Pavan Muktasana,
                                             Tadagi Mudra,
                                             Bhujangasana,
                                             Shalabhasana,
                                             Vakrasana,
                                             Gomukhasana,
                                             Vajrasana (after meal).

19. Menstrual disorders   K-   Kunjal, LSP.
                                        A-   Suryanamaskar,
                                             Sarvangasana,
                                             Bhujangasana,
                                             Shalabhasana,
                                             Dhanurasana,
                                             Matsyasana.

	P-	Kapalbhati, Anuloma-Viloma, Sheetakari, Bhramari, Yoga Nidra.
20. Obesity	K-	Kunjal, LSP.
	A-	Suryanamaskar, Uttan Padasana, Pavan Muktasana, Dhanurasana, Utthitpadasana, Janusirasana, Bhujangasana, Shalabhasana, Vakrasana.
	P-	Kapalbhati, Bhastrika, Anuloma-Viloma, Suryabhedana.
21. Ischemic Heart Disease (IHD)	A-	Ardha Halasana, Uttan Tadasana, Katichalana, Parvatasana, Shavasana.
	P-	Sukha Pranayama, lung-breathing exercises, Sheetali, Sheetakari, Yoga Nidra.
22. Weak memory	K-	Sutraneti, Jalaneti, Kunjal.
	A-	Sarvanagasana, Matsyasana, Halasana, Paschimottasana, Ardha Matsyendrasana, Ustrasana, Shirshasana, Shavasana.
	P-	Kapalbhati, Anuloma-Viloma, Bhramari, Yoga Nidra.

- **23. Height for children**

K-   Kunjal, Jalaneti.

A-   Suryanamaskara,
Matsyasana,
Suptavajrasana,
Dhanurasana,
Paschimottanasana,
Ustrasana,
Padahastasana,
Tadasana.

**24. Disorder of the male
reproductive system**

K-   Kunjal, LSP.

A-   Padmasana,
Matsyasana, Halasana,
Ustrasana,
Paschimottasana, Pada
Hastasana, Ardha-
Matsyendrasana,
Vajrasana,
Shirshasana.

P-   Kapalbhati, Bhastrika,
Anuloma-Viloma,
Bhramari.

25. Myopia

K-   Jalaneti, Steam
Inhalation.

A-   Sarvangasana,
Matsyasana,
Bhujangasana,
Shalabhasana,
Dhanurasana,
Utthitpadasana,
Simhasana,
Eye Exercises,
Shavasana.

P-   Kapalbhati, Bhastrika,
Anuloma-Viloma,
Bhramari.